Frozen Section Library

**Series Editor
Philip T. Cagle, MD
Houston, Texas, USA**

For further volumes:
http://www.springer.com/series/7869

Frozen Section Library: Gynecologic Pathology Intraoperative Consultation

by

Donna M. Coffey

*Department of Pathology and Genomic Medicine,
The Methodist Hospital, Houston, TX, USA*

Ibrahim Ramzy

*Departments of Pathology and of Obstetrics-Gynecology,
University of California, Irvine, CA, USA*

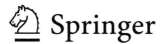

Donna M. Coffey, MD
Assistant Professor of Pathology and Laboratory Medicine
Weill Medical College of Cornell University
Department of Pathology and Genomic Medicine
The Methodist Hospital
Houston, TX 77030, USA
dcoffey@tmhs.org

Ibrahim Ramzy, MD, FRCP(C)
Professor of Pathology and of Obstetrics-Gynecology
University of California, Irvine
California 92697, USA
iramzy@uci.edu

ISSN 1868-4157　　　　　　　　e-ISSN 1868-4165
ISBN 978-0-387-95957-3　　　　 e-ISBN 978-0-387-95958-0
DOI 10.1007/978-0-387-95958-0
Springer New York Dordrecht Heidelberg London

Library of Congress Control Number: 2011939064

© Springer Science+Business Media, LLC 2012
All rights reserved. This work may not be translated or copied in whole or in part without the written permission of the publisher (Springer Science+Business Media, LLC, 233 Spring Street, New York, NY 10013, USA), except for brief excerpts in connection with reviews or scholarly analysis. Use in connection with any form of information storage and retrieval, electronic adaptation, computer software, or by similar or dissimilar methodology now known or hereafter developed is forbidden.
The use in this publication of trade names, trademarks, service marks, and similar terms, even if they are not identified as such, is not to be taken as an expression of opinion as to whether or not they are subject to proprietary rights.
While the advice and information in this book are believed to be true and accurate at the date of going to press, neither the authors nor the editors nor the publisher can accept any legal responsibility for any errors or omissions that may be made. The publisher makes no warranty, express or implied, with respect to the material contained herein.

Printed on acid-free paper

Springer is part of Springer Science+Business Media (www.springer.com)

To
Alfredo and Faye
In recognition of their unconditional love, encouragement,
and selfless support of our careers

and to our
Mentors and Students
Who continue to enrich our professional lives

Foreword

One of the closest relationships that exists in the field of medicine is that of the gynecologic pathologist and the gynecologic surgeon. The key element of this relationship is the trust that develops during the execution of a diagnosis on frozen section. The dramas of many of the situations that arise are exemplified by the following: a frozen section will be done on a conization of the uterine cervix prior to a surgical procedure for removal of the uterus. If the patient has pre-invasive disease, a simple hysterectomy will be done. If the patient has invasion to a significant degree, a radical hysterectomy will be done. The decision rests with the gynecologic pathologist and his/her diagnosis. An equally important decision might be an adnexal mass in a nulliparous woman of 22 years. The mass is submitted for frozen section and a decision as to the histology is awaited. Is the mass benign or malignant? If it is malignant, is it a borderline lesion, where conservative therapy would be very reasonable, or is it a frankly malignant lesion, where more radical surgery would be more curative? The patient's fertility and ability for future child bearing hangs in the balance. I have given these two examples to underline the important relationship that exists between the gynecologic surgeon and the pathologist executing a frozen section report. Decisions must be made in the operating room and optimum accuracy is extremely desirable.

This text reviews the critical differential diagnostic features that are crucial for the gynecologic pathologist while making these decisions. The text discusses the preparation of the specimen for frozen section and addresses the variety of specimens that arrive from the operating room. Appropriately, the limitations of intraoperative consultation by frozen section, along with the diagnostic criteria for making a diagnosis, are detailed. Doctors Coffey and Ramzy have produced a unique addition to our literature by addressing a very key procedure for clinical diagnosis. I take the privilege to suggest that it should be on the bookshelf of every gynecologic pathologist and gynecologic surgeon.

Sincerely,

Irvine, CA, USA　　　　　　　　　　　　　　　　Philip J. Di Saia, MD

Preface

Intraoperative consultation is often the cornerstone for optimizing surgical management of disease. Nowhere is this principle more evident than in the field of Gynecologic Pathology. An open and clear dialogue between the pathologist and the gynecologist is critical; it ensures that the pathologist has all the information needed to arrive at the correct interpretation of the material. For the gynecologic oncologist, it assures the best evaluation of the material and allows for clarification of any issues regarding the procedure, such as which margins are involved, and how close a tumor is from a specific margin. The value of freezing a minute specimen should be weighed against the potential of destroying it, thereby hindering the ability to establish a definitive diagnosis on permanent sections. Although the resolution of these issues needs to be documented on paper, the subtleties can only be conveyed through direct interaction, often face to face, between members of the team.

The handbook is not an attempt to cover Gynecologic Pathology in depth in an encyclopedic format; several outstanding texts are readily available for that purpose. It is designed to address practical issues, as encountered by the surgical pathologist in the daily practice of intraoperative gross and microscopic consultation. It reflects our experience in several tertiary care hospital settings with active gynecologic oncology services. The format follows a variety of specimens as they arrive at the frozen section room from the operating room, and the sequence of events that are initiated in examining, processing, and reporting the results. It highlights the ensuing dialogue between the pathologist and the gynecologist seeking specific information from the consult. To achieve that, the text is not limited to discussion of frozen sections; it encompasses all aspects of intraoperative consultation. Critical differential diagnostic issues are considered in detail, and the limitations of intraoperative consults are considered. The key features of common lesions are listed to highlight their diagnostic criteria. An ample use of figures helps to illustrate and contrast features of the different tumors encountered. Except when noted, all illustrations are from our personal files, and all histologic slides, unless stated otherwise, are stained with routine Hematoxylin and Eosin.

We would like to acknowledge the support and valuable input of many of our colleagues, both pathologists and gynecologic oncologists, with whom we have had the good fortune of working for many years at the Methodist Hospital and Baylor College of Medicine in Houston, and at the University of California Irvine. In particular, the input of Drs. Alan Kaplan and Philip DiSaia is greatly appreciated and deserves a special mention. Their wisdom, support, and critical thinking greatly contributed to our experience and are visible throughout the text.

Houston, TX, USA Donna M. Coffey, MD
Irvine, CA, USA Ibrahim Ramzy, MD

Contents

1. General Principles 1
2. Vulva 5
3. Vagina 33
4. Uterine Cervix 59
5. Uterine Body 103
6. Ovary and Fallopian Tube 153
7. Concluding Remarks 229

Index 231

Chapter 1
General Principles

Gynecologic specimens are frequently submitted for intraoperative consultation, primarily to guide the scope of surgery. The main indications for frozen section in gynecologic surgery are to aid the surgeon in determining the extent of tumor spread, locally and in lymph nodes, to confirm the diagnosis of ovarian or other malignant condition prior to radical surgery, and to ensure the adequacy of biopsy or resection.

Improved imaging techniques, as well as serology testing, help the gynecologist in making a more accurate preoperative diagnosis and determine the resectability of a lesion or possible metastatic spread. With this information, the gynecologist can plan the type and extent of the procedure. During surgery, however, the gynecologist may encounter findings that need clarification as to their nature and expected behavior, or may discover a new unexpected lesion that needs to be identified prior to proceeding with the definitive surgery. In such a scenario, close intraoperative consultation with the surgical pathologist becomes critical to ensure optimal patient care. To achieve that level of care, clinical information obtained from preoperative tests are valuable to the pathologist, who should integrate them with the gross and histomorphologic findings, thereby increasing the accuracy of frozen section interpretation. At our institution, approximately 10% of all cases submitted for intraoperative consultation and/or frozen sections are gynecologic specimens. Of these, 40% are from ovarian lesions, 40% are from uterine lesions including the cervix, and the remaining 20% are from vulvar and vaginal samples. The extent or type of surgery is often dependent on the results of such examinations. Table 1.1 lists some general and common reasons for seeking intraoperative consults,

TABLE 1.1 Reasons for requesting intraoperative consultation.

Gross consult
- Confirm the presence of a mass/lesion in resected specimen
- Establish benign versus malignant nature of a mass
- Obtain material for further tests that require fresh samples, e.g., drug sensitivity
- Procure material for microbiologic cultures and studies
- Obtain samples for immunotherapy, targeted therapy, cell cycle analysis, and tissue culture
- Procure samples for RNA and other studies that require fresh material or freezing in liquid nitrogen

Microscopic examination by frozen section
- Confirm the diagnosis of malignancy prior to resection of a mass
- Confirm the benign nature of a lesion if conservative procedures are contemplated
- Assess the status of resection margins and assess the adequacy of excision
- Assess the status of lymph nodes
- Determine the nature of a nodule discovered intraoperatively on the peritoneal surface, liver, or other organs to exclude metastases
- Establish the nature of suspicious areas in an otherwise benign-appearing cyst or mass
- Determine if the lesion is inoperable
- Map the extent of surgical resection

although reasons are often organ-specific. They also depend on the type of surgery contemplated and any unexpected findings encountered during the procedure.

Despite inherent technical difficulties in processing, sectioning, and staining of frozen sections, the technique is fairly reliable. In general surgical practice, the accuracy of frozen section is reported to vary from 91.5 to 97.4% (Wang 1998). In lesions where mitotic counts are critical, such as mesenchymal neoplasms, or where extensive sampling is necessary because of the coexistence of benign and malignant components, the accuracy drops. In such instances, it is imperative to defer the diagnosis until additional examination becomes feasible.

Frozen sections are most useful in cases where the surgical procedure is affected, such as evaluation of lymph nodes in vulvar or cervical cancer, myometrial lesions in young patients where myomectomy is considered, ovarian tumors to determine primary from secondary neoplasms, and to establish margins in vulvar or cervical tumors. Frozen sections are also valuable in endometrial carcinomas to determine prognostic factors and in suspected recurrences or metastases to determine adequacy of biopsy material.

Intraoperative consultation plays a different role in each part of the female genital tract, and the text will consider each organ separately. The application, indications, contraindications, and limitations of intraoperative gross and microscopic consultation in gynecologic specimens will be discussed, as well as causes of false frozen section results. Techniques of handling different specimens will only be considered in as much as they relate to frozen section, and gross consultation carried within the operating room suite or the frozen section laboratory.

RECOMMENDED READING

Acs G. Intraoperative consultation in gynecologic pathology. Semin Diagn Pathol. 2002;19:237–54.

American Joint Committee on Cancer. AJCC cancer staging manual. 7th ed. New York: Springer; 2010.

Baker P, Oliva E. A practical approach to intraoperative consultation in gynecological pathology. Int J Gynecol Pathol. 2008;27:353–65.

Benedet JL, Bender H, Jones 3rd H, et al. FIGO staging classifications and clinical practice guidelines in the management of gynecologic cancers. FIGO Committee on Gynecologic Oncology. Int J Gynecol Obstet. 2000; 70:209–62.

Berek JS, Hacker NF, editors. Berek & Hacker's practical gynecologic oncology. 5th ed. Philadelphia, PA: Lippincott Williams & Wilkins; 2009.

Clements PB, Young RH. Atlas of gynecologic surgical pathology. Philadelphia, PA: WB Saunders; 2000.

Crum CP, Lee KR, editors. Diagnostic gynecologic and obstetric pathology. Philadelphia, PA: Elsevier Saunders; 2006.

DiSaia PJ, Creasman WT. Clinical gynecologic oncology. 7th ed. Philadelphia, PA: Mosby-Elsevier; 2007.

Hoskins W, Perez CA, Young RC. Principles and practice of gynecologic oncology. 3rd ed. Philadelphia, PA: Lippincott William and Wilkins; 2000.

Ismiil N, Ghorab Z, Nofech-Mozes S, et al. Intraoperative consultation in gynecologic pathology: a 6 year audit at a tertiary care medical center. Int J Gynecol Cancer. 2009;19:152–7.

Nucci MR, Oliva E, editors. Gynecologic pathology a volume in the series foundations in diagnostic pathology. London: Elsevier Churchill Livingstone; 2009.

Rock JA, Johns III HW. TeLinde's operative gynecology. 10th ed. Philadelphia, PA: Lippincott; 2008.

Robboy SJ, Anderson MC, Russell P, editors. Pathology of the female reproductive tract. London: Churchill Livingstone; 2002.

Saglam EA, Usubutum A, Ayhan A, et al. Mistakes prevent mistakes: experience from intraoperative consultation with frozen section. Eur J Obstet Gynecol Reprod Biol. 2006;125:266–8.

Wang KG, Chen TC, Wang TY, et al. Accuracy of frozen section diagnosis in gynecology. Gynecol Oncol. 1998;70:105–10.

Chapter 2
Vulva

Benign and malignant neoplasms as well as reactive inflammatory lesions of the vulva present as ulcers, white plaques, swellings, and red or dark pigmented lesions. In view of the overlap in clinical and gross features, surgical sampling is often required to establish the diagnosis. Almost all intraoperative consultations relate to the evaluation of malignant or premalignant lesions (Table 2.1). Specimens generally fall into two categories: (a) biopsies and other limited procedures for diagnostic/therapeutic indications and (b) a variety of vulvar resections of pre-neoplastic and neoplastic lesions.

VULVAR BIOPSIES AND OTHER LIMITED PROCEDURES

Clinical Background and Specimen Handling
Small biopsies are performed either as diagnostic procedures for a suspicious area such as hyperkeratosis, or as simple local excisions of a benign solid lesion or a cyst. Biopsies are not usually submitted for immediate interpretation except under unusual circumstances, since the results of frozen sections will not change the immediate management. The biopsy should be properly oriented on a firm surface with the epidermal surface up to keep the specimen as flat as possible for examination or fixation in the laboratory (Fig. 2.1).

Other limited treatment or biopsy modalities used in vulvar disease include cryosurgery, laser surgery, electrocautery, and 5-fluorouracil. These are used for the treatment of small lesions, particularly when conservative therapy is indicated. Such specimens are not submitted for intraoperative consultation. They are not usually suitable for histopathologic evaluation in view of the complete destruction of tissues or the marked artifactual changes that preclude proper examination.

TABLE 2.1 Reasons for intraoperative consultation in vulvar lesions.

- Determine the presence and depth of invasive component
- Determine the adequacy of resection by examining the surgical margins
- Establish the status of pelvic lymph nodes
- Exclude the presence of peritoneal spread
- Differentiate primary from metastatic malignancies

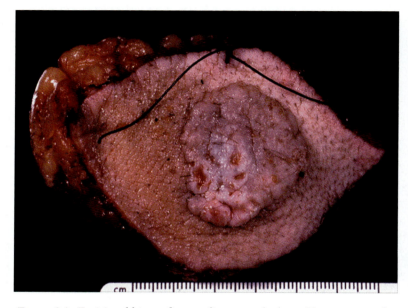

FIGURE 2.1 Excisional biopsy for a malignant melanoma. The suture marks the lateral margin of resection.

Interpretation and Limitations

The most critical role of intraoperative consultation in the vulva is to rule out malignancy and map the extent of resection in the context of a vulvectomy for cancer, as discussed below. Non-neoplastic epithelial disorders of vulvar skin and mucosa such as squamous cell hyperplasia, lichen sclerosus, and other dermatoses are some of the lesions that may be encountered in such a scenario, and may raise differential diagnostic issues. An adequate biopsy should include the epidermis and at least the superficial dermis. A rim of normal tissue can be helpful in identifying early changes that may be masked by necrosis or inflammatory exudate in the center of the sample. Freezing artifacts also interfere with the ability to arrive at a diagnosis on subsequent permanent sections. In small lesions that were completely excised, trimming to "face" the biopsy risks loss of tissue at the edge of the blade, thus permanently missing any chance to establish the nature of the lesion. Pressure to make a hasty diagnosis, in the absence of a good reason, should be resisted, since it can be a disservice to the patient.

VULVECTOMY FOR SQUAMOUS CELL CANCER

Cancer of the vulva comprises only 5% of all gynecologic malignancies. It predominantly affects postmenopausal women. The majority of malignancies arise within the squamous epithelium, most commonly on the labia majora, labia minora, clitoris, and perineum. Studies suggest that there are two etiologic types of vulvar cancer. One type is the warty or basaloid carcinomas that are seen in younger patients; these are related to human papilloma virus (HPV) and are associated with warty or basaloid vulvar intraepithelial neoplasia (VIN). The second type, keratinizing squamous cell carcinoma seen in elderly patients, is unrelated to HPV infection and is associated with differentiated (simplex) VIN. These patients have a high incidence of lichen sclerosus adjacent to the neoplasm.

Clinical Background and Specimen Types

The modern approach to the management of patients with carcinoma confined to the vulva should be individualized. Emphasis is on performing the most conservative operation consistent with cure of the disease. Several types of vulvectomy are tailored to treat squamous cell carcinoma, depending on the location, type, and extent of the tumor, stage of disease, and other clinical parameters such as risk tolerance. Wide local excision (disease-free border of at least 5 mm) is performed for the treatment of premalignant lesions or minimally invasive cancer. Partial or total vulvectomy is usually performed for invasive cancers, with inclusion of a portion of the vagina and extensions of perineum around the anus in some cases (Fig. 2.2). The depth of resection may be variable. In skinning vulvectomy, the epidermis and a variable amount of dermis are included. Radical vulvectomy is a more extensive procedure that is less frequently performed. It involves resection of the superficial aponeurosis of the urogenital diaphragm and/or pubic periosteum in addition to the vulva proper (Fig. 2.3). Pelvic exenteration, combined with radical vulvectomy, is rarely used for the treatment of vulvar cancer, and is limited to exceptional cases with the involvement of the anus, rectovaginal septum, or proximal urethra. It includes resection of several pelvic organs. Inguinal lymph nodes may also be resected for vulvar malignancies. Since the lymphatics drain primarily into

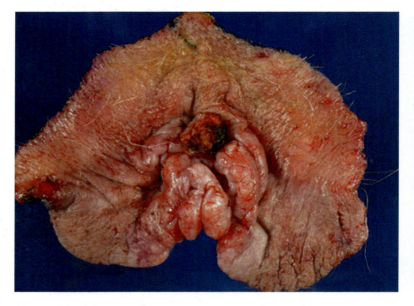

FIGURE 2.2 Vulvectomy for carcinoma in situ. The neoplastic process may be multifocal and bilateral, thus determining the extent of the surgery.

the superficial and deep (femoral) inguinal nodes, both levels of nodes are usually resected in cases of carcinoma.

Specimen Handling

The initial laboratory evaluation of any vulvar excision must include orientation of the specimen as if viewed in situ. Orientation by the surgeon is critical if the adequacy of the resection is to be assessed. Photographs and diagrams/drawings to demonstrate the margins of resection and extent of the lesion are also helpful. Deep margins should be inked, and different colors should be used for vaginal tissue or any margin toward the anal canal (Figs. 2.4 and 2.5). Margins that are macroscopically close to the tumor are preferably evaluated with sections that are perpendicular, rather than parallel, to the surgical margin. Other margins that are distant to the lesion can be evaluated with sections parallel to the margin. This approach will reduce the number of sections, intraoperative consultation time, as well as the overall operating time. In many instances, the status of the deep soft tissue margin can be assessed macroscopically. Microscopic examination of the deep margins is recommended if, on gross examination, the tumor approaches the deep soft tissue margin. The frozen section report should include the size and location of

VULVA 9

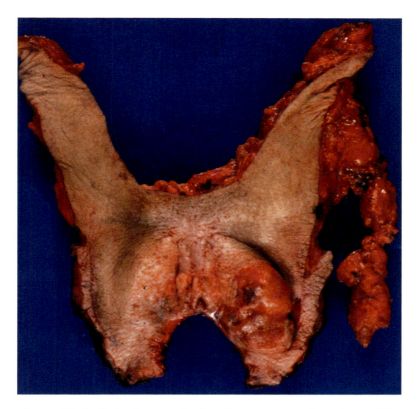

FIGURE 2.3 Radical vulvectomy for invasive squamous cell carcinoma. The vulva, part of inguinal skin, and soft tissues, as well as lymph nodes are included in this specimen.

the lesion, status of the cutaneous and mucosal margins, and status of the deep margin as well as the maximum depth of invasion.

Interpretation and Differential Diagnostic Considerations
Squamous cell carcinoma and its intraepithelial precursors are the most common malignant neoplasms of vulva, with invasive lesions accounting for about 90% of all vulvar cancers and about 5% of all gynecologic cancers. The role of the human papilloma virus in the pathogenesis of this tumor has been well documented, but a detailed discussion is beyond the scope of this text. The neoplastic process encompasses a spectrum of morphologic changes, ranging from mild cytologic atypia in intraepithelial lesions to high-grade invasive carcinomas.

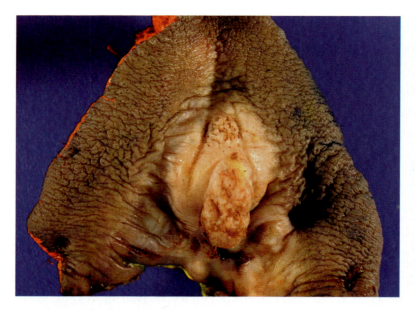

FIGURE 2.4 Vulvectomy for squamous cell carcinoma to demonstrate the inking of the resection margins using different colors.

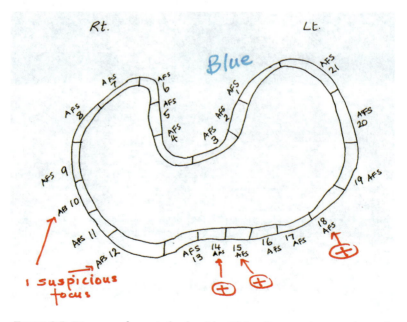

FIGURE 2.5 Diagram of resected vulva, identifying the resection margins and location of each section can be critical in assessing the margins.

VULVA 11

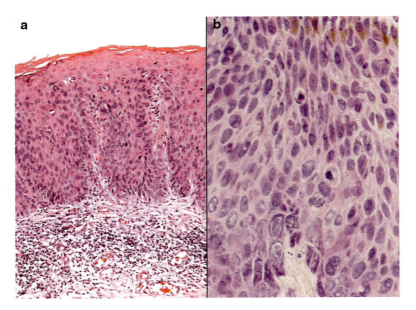

FIGURE 2.6 Vulvar intraepithelial neoplasia (VIN III): (**a**) Involvement of the entire thickness of the squamous epithelium by the atypical cells. Surface keratinization is evident and the dermis is infiltrated by chronic inflammatory cells (H&E, medium power). (**b**) Higher magnification shows nuclear pleomorphism and dyspolarity in the entire thickness of the epithelium.

Vulvar Intraepithelial Neoplasia

Frozen sections should not be performed solely to evaluate the grade of vulvar intraepithelial neoplasia (VIN). However, they are necessary for the assessment of margins to exclude any high-grade VIN, in view of the increased risk of recurrence or progression to invasive disease (Fig. 2.6). Adjacent foci of VIN or hyperplasia with or without atypia are seen in many cases of invasive squamous cell carcinoma (Fig. 2.7). In cases with superficially invasive carcinomas, the frequency of adjacent VIN approaches 85% (Hoskins 2000). A thorough evaluation of all the margins in large vulvar resections is only feasible on permanent sections. Multifocal high-grade dysplasia often presents a challenge, in view of the difficulty in obtaining a clear resection margin. Foci of unsuspected invasion may occur in up to 19% of patients with VIN (Chafe 1998). In evaluating the presence and depth of invasion, involvement of adnexal structures by VIN should not be considered evidence of invasion

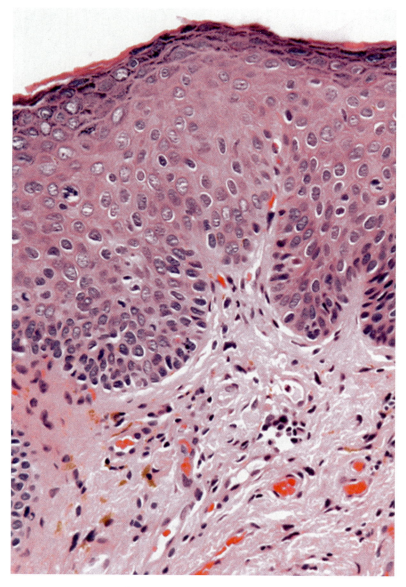

FIGURE 2.7 Vulvar intraepithelial neoplasia (VIN III) and hyperplasia with atypia, seen at the margin of an invasive tumor (H&E, medium power).

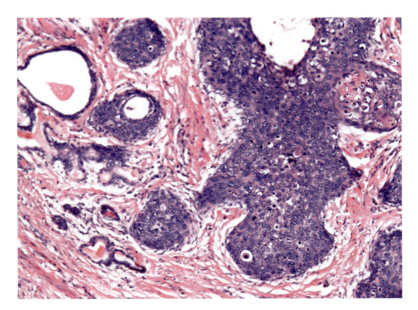

FIGURE 2.8 VIN III in Bartholin duct: The patient had an extensive multifocal VIN III of the surface epithelium that extended into the Bartholin duct. The neoplasia remains confined within the basement membrane of the duct and should not be considered evidence of invasive disease, despite the deep location of the lesion (H&E, medium power).

(Fig. 2.8). Similarly, any tangential sectioning of the VIN lesion should not be misinterpreted. Evidence of a residual appendage, lack of a desmoplastic stromal response, and presence of circumscribed, rather than irregular, borders help in differentiating this artifact from true stromal invasion (Fig. 2.9). Sectioning the frozen tissue at more than one level can also resolve this issue.

Vulvar intraepithelial neoplasia is frequently associated with similar lesions in other pelvic organs. Approximately 50–60% of women with VIN who exhibit evidence of HPV infection have similar synchronous or metachronous lesions in the cervix, vagina, urethra, perineum, or anus. If these areas are included with the resection, they should be sampled extensively, at the time the specimen is processed, for routine microscopic examination.

Invasive Squamous Cell Carcinomas
Vulvar squamous cell carcinomas are often well differentiated neoplasms, with evidence of keratinization (Fig. 2.10). If they ulcerate, the stroma shows a mixture of acute and chronic inflammatory

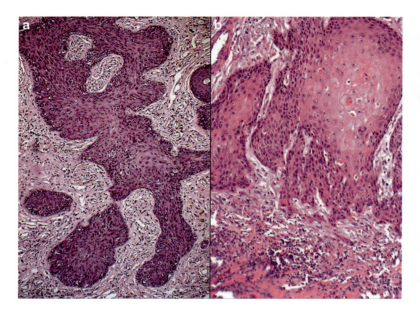

FIGURE 2.9 (**a**) VIN III showing tangential cutting. The presence of islands of stroma within the epithelium, rounded margins of the epithelial nests, and lack of stromal inflammatory or desmoplastic response speak against true invasion. (**b**) Invasive squamous carcinoma, for comparison. This section from the margin of a vulvectomy reveals that the invading columns of neoplastic cells are irregular, pointed, and induce a stromal reaction (H&E, medium power).

cellular response (Fig. 2.11). Assessment of the vascular spread can be difficult at the time of intraoperative consultation. Freezing or fixation artifacts may result in the separation of nests of tumor cells from the surrounding connective tissue. Such retraction, however, is usually incomplete, leaving some parts of the tumor attached to the wall. Immunostains for endothelial markers may be necessary to settle the issue on permanent sections (Fig. 2.12). The management of invasive tumors varies with the stage and extent of the lesion. In FIGO stage IA, the tumor measures 2 cm or less, with 0.1 cm or less depth of invasion, and is associated with clinically negative nodes. These lesions tend to affect younger women and are commonly associated with multifocal pre-invasive disease and evidence of HPV infection. Such patients have a high risk of recurrence or development of new lesions. Wide local or superficial local excisions that incorporate a 1 cm normal tissue margin are the usual

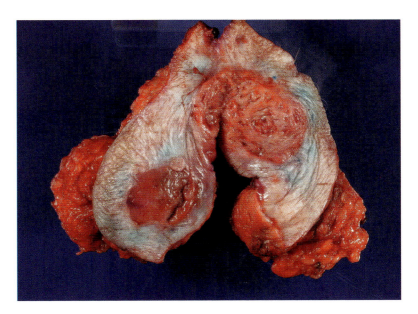

FIGURE 2.10 Invasive squamous cell carcinoma. The tumor involves both sides of the vulva. The *left side* lesion is ulcerated and involves midline structures.

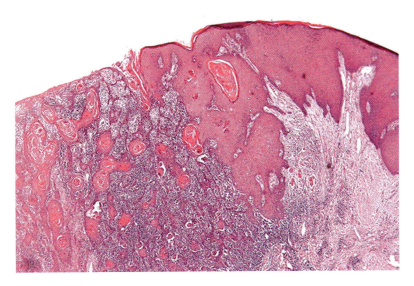

FIGURE 2.11 Invasive squamous cell carcinoma. A well differentiated tumor, showing surface ulceration with intense inflammatory reaction in the stroma.

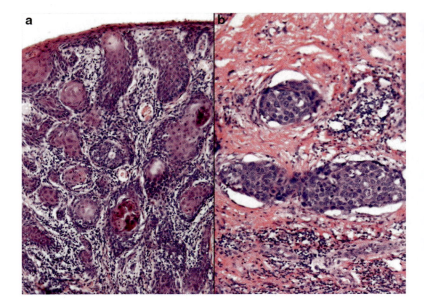

FIGURE 2.12 Invasive squamous cell carcinoma. (**a**) A well differentiated keratinizing squamous cell carcinoma with stromal inflammatory response. (**b**) Shrinkage fixation artifact partially separates nests of tumor cells from the surrounding stroma. Unlike true vascular invasion, the neoplastic cells are partially attached to the stroma and the nests lack a *round* or *oval shape* with a smooth margin. In problematic cases, immunostains for endothelial markers will clarify the issue (H&E, medium power).

treatment modality for such tumors. The incidence of local invasive recurrence is low if the margin is at least 0.8 cm.

For stage IB and II vulvar cancers, the usual management is radical local excision with unilateral or bilateral inguinal node dissection, contingent upon whether the lesion is laterally located or in the midline. This approach provides long-term survival, but has significant morbidity. More recent emphasis has been placed on developing individualized treatment, with limited resections for certain subsets considered to represent early or low-risk disease. In stage IB carcinoma, for example, a more conservative resection of the primary tumor with a 1–2 cm margin of normal tissue, and dissection to the deep perineal fascia, combined with inguinal lymph node dissection, is currently recommended.

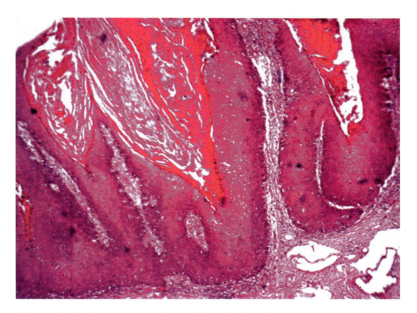

FIGURE 2.13 Verrucous carcinoma. This highly differentiated squamous cell carcinoma is often treated by wide local excision. The neoplastic epithelium extends deeply into the subepithelial tissues by bulbous nests that have a pushing, rather than infiltrating, border. There is marked hyperkeratosis as well as parakeratosis. Unlike warty invasive carcinoma, the cytologic atypia is minimal, and the lesion is often interpreted as hyperplasia in the initial biopsies (H&E, medium power).

Verrucous Carcinoma

This uncommon, highly differentiated squamous cell carcinoma has been associated with HPV serotypes 1, 2, 6, 11, 16, and 18. Verrucous carcinoma has a tendency to involve a few specific areas, including the vulva, oral cavity, and larynx. It is a low-grade, locally invasive neoplasm that rarely metastasizes and has excellent prognosis. Consequently, treatment by a wide local excision is usually curative. The tumor has a tendency for local recurrences, especially if it has been incompletely resected. Intraoperative evaluation of these cases includes gross inspection of the lesion and its relationship to the margins of resection. Frozen section of grossly or clinically suspicious margins can be performed, and, since deep pushing penetration by bulbous epithelial masses with deep keratinization is a helpful feature, the pathologist should not hesitate in asking for deep excisions to assess the relationship with the dermis (Fig. 2.13).

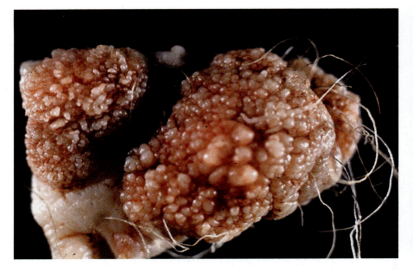

FIGURE 2.14 Condyloma acuminatum: These are often multiple, flesh colored, and may involve other areas of the perineum. When they are extensive and single, the possibility of verrucous carcinoma should be considered. The differentiation can be difficult, and the implication of over-treating a condyloma versus under-treating a carcinoma is quite significant, particularly in young patients. From Ramzy I: Essentials of Gynecologic and Obstetric Pathology, p.49. Norwalk: Appleton Century Crofts, 1983. Used with permission.

Verrucous carcinomas should be differentiated from warty invasive squamous cell carcinoma and condyloma acuminatum. Invasive warty squamous cell carcinomas have a significant degree of atypia and an infiltrative border, unlike the minimal cytologic atypia and mostly pushing borders that characterize verrucous carcinomas. Condylomas lack the deep penetration by bulbous growth and keratinization at the base that are seen in verrucous carcinoma (Figs. 2.14 and 2.15).

Differential Diagnosis of Verrucous Lesions

Key Histologic Features of Verrucous Carcinoma
- Bulbous nests of neoplastic cells with pushing border
- Tumor cells have abundant cytoplasm with minimal atypia
- Hyperplastic squamous epithelium
- Prominent hyperkeratosis and parakeratosis

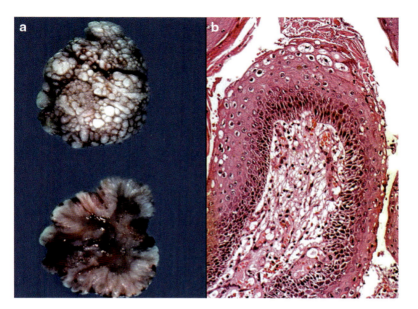

FIGURE 2.15 Condyloma acuminatum: (**a**) The outer surface and the cut section reveal the verrucous appearance of the lesion. (**b**) There is papillary proliferation, acanthosis, and hyperkeratosis. Koilocytosis is evident, particularly near the surface. The vascular stroma has a few inflammatory cells (H&E, medium power).

Key Histologic Features of Warty (Condylomatous) Carcinoma
- Papillae lined by squamous epithelium with koilocytic change on the surface
- Significant cytologic atypia, and deep keratinization at the base and in the invasive nests
- Infiltrative-jagged borders

Key Features of Condyloma Acuminatum
- Papillary architecture
- Acanthotic squamous epithelium with hyperkeratosis, parakeratosis, and hypergranulosis
- Koilocytic atypia on the surface
- No pushing border or infiltrative border

LYMPH NODE DISSECTION IN VULVAR CANCER

This is usually indicated in patients with more than 1 mm stromal invasion. The resection may be unilateral or bilateral, depending on the location and extent of the malignancy. Sentinel lymph node evaluation in vulvar carcinomas is a feasible technique that can be utilized to reduce complications and morbidity associated with inguinofemoral lymphadenectomy.

The inguinal node component can be attached to the vulvar resection or submitted separately. The superficial inguinal nodes are the most common sites of metastasis. Nodal involvement generally proceeds in a stepwise fashion from superficial to deep inguinal nodes and then to the pelvic (iliac) nodes (Fig. 2.16).

Tumor involvement of pelvic lymph nodes including internal iliac, external iliac, and common iliac lymph nodes is considered distant metastasis. Surgical resection of deep inguinal or femoral lymph nodes is usually performed in conjunction with superficial inguinal lymphadenectomy. In most cases, these samples are submitted independently from the vulvar specimen. Frozen section is not usually requested for node dissections since the results rarely have an impact on the immediate operative management. In the rare instances where an intraoperative consultation on a node is required, the initial evaluation must include a count of lymph nodes identified and the gross inspection of the cut surface. In cases where sentinel lymph node or Cloquet lymph node evaluation is requested, the entire node(s) should be submitted for frozen section. Touch imprints of the cut surface assist in the initial evaluation of metastatic disease. Areas of firmness or variation in color should raise suspicion of involvement by metastatic disease, and such areas should be selected for frozen sections, if necessary. Frozen section diagnosis, however, can be difficult in cases where only few atypical cells are noted, and, if immediate management is not altered by lymph nodes status, evaluation should be deferred until permanent sections are examined.

VULVECTOMY FOR OTHER MALIGNANCIES

Rare malignancies that may be encountered include malignant melanoma, Paget disease, adenocarcinomas, and basal cell carcinoma. Soft tissue sarcomas, such as leiomyosarcoma, angiosarcoma, liposarcoma, or embryonal rhabdomyosarcoma, are rarely seen in the vulva. In addition, metastatic tumors from other genital organs can appear in the vulvar skin or mucosa.

Malignant Melanoma

This is the second most common vulvar malignancy, usually involving the labia majora, labia minora, clitoris, and perineum, in

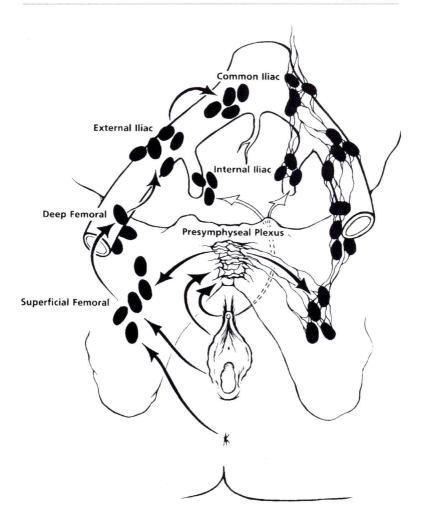

FIGURE 2.16 Lymphatic drainage of vulva. From: Ramzy I, Vulvar lesions and pruritus. In Pauerstein, CJ: Gynecologic Disorders, Differential diagnosis and therapy. 1982, Grune & Stratton, New York, NY, p 313. Used with permission.

descending order. The main treatment modality is surgical resection. Melanoma in situ is usually treated with complete excision of the gross lesion, the full thickness of the underlying dermis, and at least a 0.5 cm rim of normal tissue. Invasive melanomas less than 0.1 cm thick are similarly managed, but with a wide (1 cm) margin,

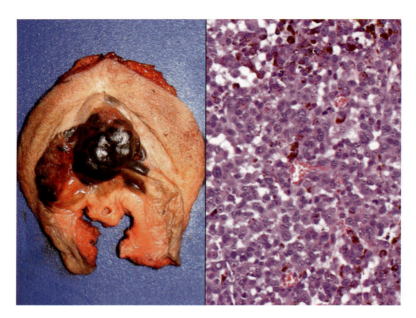

FIGURE 2.17 Malignant melanoma: (**a**) A large mass involving the midline and both sides of the anterior vulva. There is dark pigmentation as well as surface ulceration and evidence of bleeding. (**b**) The frozen section reveals neoplastic cells infiltrating deeply into the dermis. Note the presence of nuclear pleomorphism, prominent nucleoli, and presence of brown melanin pigmentation (H&E, medium power).

although the utility of such wider margins for deeper melanomas is debatable (see Fig. 2.1). Radical vulvectomy with lymph node dissection is necessary in large melanomas, or for those tumors involving the urethra, clitoris, or lower vagina (Figs. 2.17 and 2.18). Sentinel lymph node evaluation is performed for tumors 0.1 cm or greater in thickness, or for melanomas with Clark level 4 or deeper, with the decision regarding lymphadenectomy based on the status of the sentinel lymph node. As in other skin sites, frozen section evaluation of margins in pigmented lesions or known melanomas is not recommended due to the difficulty of interpretation with freezing artifact and the ensuing cytoplasmic vacuolization. These artifactual changes can be misinterpreted as involvement by atypical melanocytes in the frozen section material, as well as in the permanent section of previously frozen tissue.

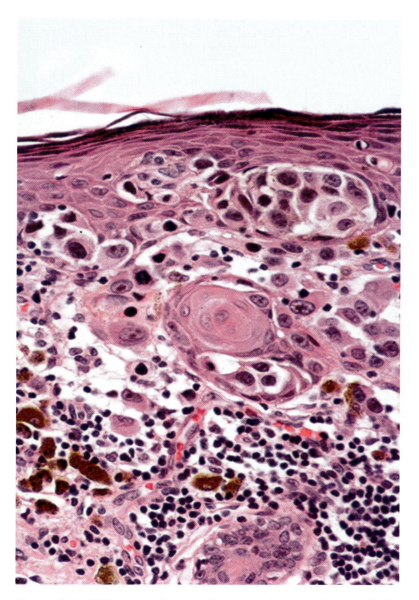

FIGURE 2.18 Malignant melanoma: Multinucleation, prominent nucleoli, intranuclear cytoplasmic inclusions, and the presence of melanin pigment help to differentiate this tumor from squamous cell carcinoma and Paget disease. Occasionally, immunostains may be necessary to confirm the diagnosis, particularly in amelanotic melanomas (H&E, medium power).

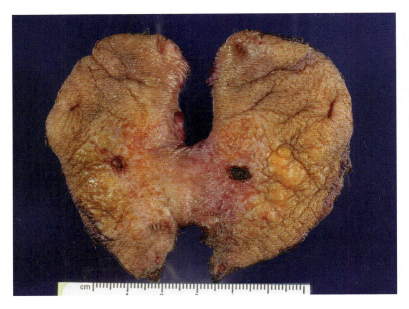

FIGURE 2.19 Paget disease: The erythematous patch shows islands of pale epithelium and foci of superficial erosion. The two areas covered with a crust are the result of biopsies to determine the extent of the lesion. Paget disease can be deceptive in its gross appearance, and frozen sections are critical in determining the extent of the lesion and the resection necessary to treat it.

Differential Diagnostic Considerations

Nevocellular nevi are not uncommon in the vulva, particularly on the labia majora. These lesions occasionally have a verrucous appearance. Unlike malignant melanomas, these benign lesions lack nuclear atypia, mitotic figures, lymphocytic, or desmoplastic reaction. Frozen sections are not appropriate to establish the diagnosis in such cases since freezing artifacts can render evaluation extremely difficult.

Extramammary Paget Disease

This uncommon disease accounts for 1% of vulvar cancers. Paget disease of the vulva, unlike its mammary counterpart, is usually a noninvasive intraepithelial lesion that can remain unchanged for many years, and it has a low potential to progress to invasive cancer (Figs. 2.19 and 2.20). Underlying invasive carcinoma is

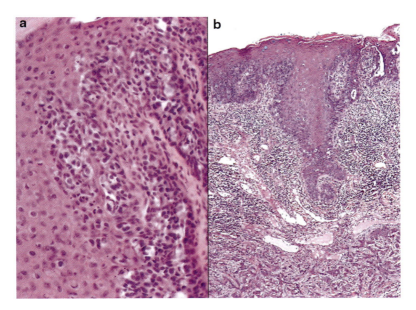

FIGURE 2.20 Paget disease: (**a**) Frozen section showing hypercellular epidermis. The differentiation from squamous cell neoplasia can be difficult in some cases. However, the presence of an occasional cell with clear cytoplasm points to Paget disease (H&E, medium power). (**b**) Paget disease with nests and cords of adenocarcinoma cells infiltrating deeply into the vulvar tissues (H&E, medium power).

identified in approximately 20% of cases. The sites of origin of the invasive component include colon/rectum cervix, bladder, or urethra. Patients with only superficial Paget disease are treated with a more conservative surgery such as local excision or skinning vulvectomy, with evaluation of the margins by frozen section. Patients with Paget disease and primary adenocarcinoma of the underlying apocrine glands are treated with radical vulvectomy and inguinal lymphadenectomy.

Differential Diagnostic Considerations
Differentiating Paget disease from pagetoid VIN and superficial spreading malignant melanoma can be extremely difficult. In pagetoid VIN, the squamous cells in the background are dysplastic, while they appear less atypical in Paget disease or in superficial spreading melanoma (Fig. 2.21). In difficult cases, the application of a

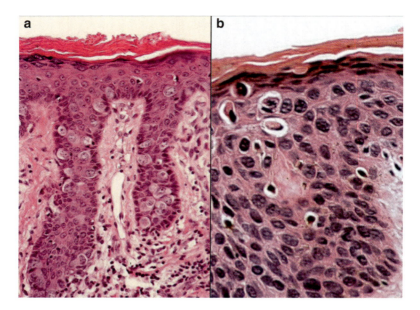

FIGURE 2.21 Paget disease versus Bowen disease (VIN III): (**a**) Paget disease showing large cells with abundant clear cytoplasm, *round* to *oval* nuclei with prominent nucleoli, in a background of normal squamous cells. (**b**) VIN III (Bowen disease) showing occasional cell within clear spaces that can simulate Paget cells, particularly on thick frozen sections. However, clear areas are around the dyskeratotic cells, not within their cytoplasm. The background squamous epithelium shows nuclear atypia (H&E, medium power). From Ramzy, I: Essentials of Gynecologic and Obstetric Pathology, p.51. Norwalk: Appleton Century Crofts, 1983. Used with permission.

modified rapid periodic-acid Schiff procedure (PAS) can be useful in identifying characteristic Paget cells with their PAS-positive vacuoles. The cells also stain positively for neutral and acidic mucin (mucicarmine, Alcian blue, and Colloidal iron) and are reactive with CEA, EMA, GCDFP, and CK7. Table 2.2 summarizes the salient features differentiating vulvar intraepithelial malignancies.

Primary Adenocarcinoma

Most vulvar adenocarcinomas are deep lesions, arising within the Bartholin gland or skin appendages. In most cases, the diagnosis has been previously established with a biopsy of the lesion

TABLE 2.2 Vulvar intraepithelial malignancies.

VIN III	Paget disease	Malignant melanoma
Clinical and gross		
Maculopapular	Eczema, ulcer or erythematous lesion	May be amelanotic or arise in nevus
White or erythematous		
May be parakeratotic	Focal white keratosis	Flat, speckled or pigmented
Neoplastic cells		
Squamous	Glandular and adnexa	Dermoepidermoid junction
Full thickness	Sq cells NL	Some pigmented
Special stains		
PAS diastase-labile	PAS diastase resistant	PAS diastase resistant
	Mucicarmine+	S 100, Dopa oxidase+
	Alcian blue+, GCDP-15+	Melan A+
	CEA+	

prior to definitive surgical resection. Approximately 20–30% have metastatic disease of the inguinal/femoral lymph nodes at time of initial diagnosis. Treatment includes a complete surgical resection and inguinal lymphadenectomy. Some benign tumors and ulcers can resemble adenocarcinoma clinically. These are discussed below. Features that suggest an adenocarcinoma include irregular infiltrating margins, desmoplastic response of the stroma, cytologic atypia, mitotic activity, and necrosis of neoplastic cells (Fig. 2.22).

Differential Diagnostic Considerations

Primary vulvar adenocarcinoma should be differentiated from metastatic adenocarcinoma, particularly of the cervix, endometrium, breast, and ovary (see below). In addition, a wide variety of benign lesions develop in the vulvar skin, adnexa, and soft tissues. Although a detailed discussion of these is beyond the scope of this text, a few lesions will be considered in view of their potential to be misinterpreted as malignancies in the frozen section room. These include papillary hidradenoma, rare cases of adenosis, hyperplasia of Bartholin glands, ectopic breast tissue, and endometriosis.

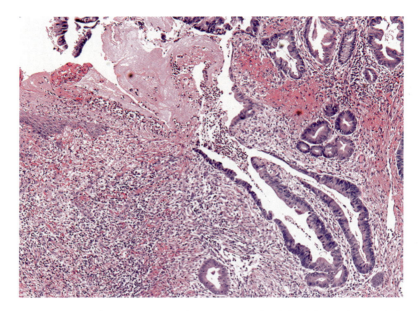

FIGURE 2.22 Adenocarcinoma: This tumor involved the vulva and extended into the lower vagina. It has ulcerated through the vulvar skin. Spread from neighboring structures such as rectum or uterus should be excluded in such cases (H&E, medium power).

Papillary hidradenoma is a benign adnexal tumor of apocrine sweat glands that may be clinically alarming because of ulceration, bleeding, or infection. It usually forms a gray or brown 1–2 cm nodule in the labium major. The tumor consists of folded papillae, clefts, and glandular spaces surrounded by a pseudocapsule. Unlike adenocarcinoma, these spaces are lined by two layers of uniform neoplastic cells: an inner cuboidal with clear PAS positive cytoplasm and a basal layer of oval myoepithelial cells that are reactive to S-100. The uniformity of the cells and the double layer of epithelium should help in differentiating this tumor from adenocarcinoma (Fig. 2.23).

Vulvar endometriosis can be easily differentiated on the basis of clinical presentation, history, and location, such as in an episiotomy scar. Occasionally, it is submitted for identification when encountered as an incidental finding during surgery.

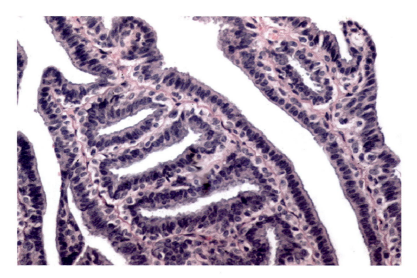

FIGURE 2.23 Hidradenoma papilliferum: The glandular spaces are lined by an inner layer of cuboidal to low columnar epithelium, and an outer layer of myoepithelial cells with relatively clear cytoplasm (H&E, medium power). From Ramzy I: Essentials of Gynecologic and Obstetric Pathology, p.39. Norwalk: Appleton Century Crofts, 1983. Used with permission.

Basal Cell Carcinoma

Only 2–3% of vulvar carcinomas are of the basal cell type, and they typically occur in elderly patients. Basal cell carcinomas are cured by wide local excisions (Fig. 2.24). When these tumors lack a clear histomorphology, such as peripheral palisading, their differentiation from Merkel-cell carcinomas, poorly differentiated squamous cell carcinomas, and metastatic small cell carcinomas may require immunostaining of permanent sections. Basal cell carcinoma should not be confused with tangentially cut basal areas of the more common squamous VIN lesions. Proper orientation of the tissue and serial sectioning should clarify this difficulty.

Metastatic Neoplasms

Metastatic tumors to the vulva are rare and occur most often in postmenopausal women. The most common source of metastases to the vulva is the genital tract, particularly the cervix, vagina,

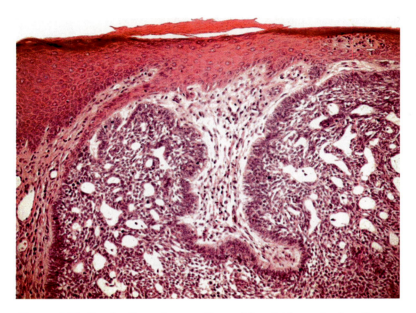

FIGURE 2.24 Basal cell carcinoma. Nests of basaloid neoplastic cells are separated by fibrous tissue bands. The basal cells are arranged in a palisading picket-fence orientation (H&E, medium power).

endometrium, and ovary. Other nongynecologic sources reported include breast, lung, kidney, colon/rectum, cutaneous melanoma, lymphomas, and genitourinary primaries. Clinical history, a review of any available material from the primary site, and additional studies using special stains and immunoprofile should establish the source in these cases.

RECOMMENDED READING

Adib T, Barton DPJ. The sentinel lymph node: relevance in gynecological cancers. Eur J Surg Oncol. 2006;32:866–74.

Ali A, Husnu C, Polat D. Lymphatic mapping and sentinel node biopsy in gynecological cancers: a critical review of the literature. World J Surg Oncol. 2008;6:53.

Bergen S, Disaia PJ, Liao SY, Berman ML. Conservative management of extramammary Paget's disease of the vulva. Gynecol Oncol. 1989; 33:151–6.

Brunner AH, Polterauer S, Tempfer C, et al. The Accuracy of intraoperative frozen section of the inguinal sentinel lymph node in vulvar cancer. Anticancer Res. 2008;28(6B):4091–4.

Chafe W, Richards A, Morgan L, et al. Unrecognized invasive carcinoma in vulvar intraepithelial neoplasia (VIN). Gynecol Oncol. 1998;31:154–65.

Chan JK, Sugiyama V, Pham H, et al. Margin distance and other clinicopathologic prognostic factors in vulvar carcinoma: a multivariate analysis. Gynecol Oncol. 2007;104:636–41.

Curtin JP, Rubin SC, Jones WB, Hoskins WJ, Lewis Jr JL. Paget's disease of the vulva. Gynecol Oncol. 1990;39:374–7.

Fishman A et al. A 30s PAS stain for frozen section analysis of surgical margins of vulvectomy in Paget's disease. Eur J Gynaecol Oncol. 1998; 19:482–3.

Gadducci A, Cionini L, Romanini A, et al. Old and new perspectives in the management of high risk, locally advanced or recurrent and metastatic vulvar cancer. Crit Rev Oncol Hematol. 2006;60:227–41.

Glass FL, Cottam JA, Reintgen DS, et al. Lymphatic mapping and sentinel node biopsy in the management of high-risk melanoma. J Am Acad Dermatol. 1998;39:603–10.

Hording U, Daugaard S, Junge J, Lundvall F. Human Papillomaviruses and multifocal genital neoplasia. Int J Gynecol Pathol. 1996;15:230–4.

Hoskins W, Perez CA, Young RC. Principles and practice of gynecologic oncology. 3rd ed. Philadelphia, PA: Lippincott, William and Wilkins; 2000.

Lars-Christian H, Wagner S. Frozen section analysis of vulvectomy specimens: results of a 5 year study period. Int J Gynecol Pathol. 2010;29:165–72.

McCluggage WG. Recent developments in vulvovaginal pathology. Histopathology. 2009;54:156–73.

Rodolakis A, Diakomanolis E, Vlachos G, et al. Vulvar intraepithelial neoplasia (VIN) – diagnostic and therapeutic challenges. Eur J Gynaecol Oncol. 2003;24:317–22.

Staats PN, Clement PB, Young RH. Primary endometrioid adenocarcinoma of the vagina: a clinicopathologic study of 18 cases. Am J Surg Pathol. 2007;10:1490–501.

Wilkinson EJ. Protocol for the examination of specimens from patients with carcinomas and malignant melanomas of the vulva: a basis for checklists. Cancer Committee of the American College of Pathologist. Arch Pathol Lab Med. 2000;124:51–6.

Chapter 3
Vagina

The majority of intraoperative consultations related to vaginal samples are to check adequacy of resection of tumors. Primary vaginal malignancies are rare; most of the intraoperative consults are for metastatic tumors that are responsible for 80% of all vaginal malignancies. Approximately a third of the metastases are of cervical origin, a fifth from the endometrium, and the remainder originates from other sites, particularly ovary, breast, and kidney. They spread to the vagina by direct extension from surrounding organs, or via lymphatic and blood vessels, most frequently involving the posterior wall of the upper third. Occasionally, pathologists are asked to identify vaginal lesions detected incidentally during other procedures or to rule out metastases. Portions of the vagina may also be included in radical resections for malignancies in other parts of the genital tract, and these will be considered with their corresponding organs (Chaps. 4–6). The present discussion will focus on lesions that primarily involve the vagina.

VAGINECTOMY FOR SQUAMOUS CELL NEOPLASMS

Clinical Background

Primary vaginal malignancies are rare, representing only 1–2% of all gynecologic cancers. Of these primary tumors, 85–90% are squamous cell carcinomas; the remainder being adenocarcinomas, clear cell carcinomas, sarcomas, and other rare lesions.

Squamous neoplasia of the vagina shares several pathogenetic and morphologic characteristics with squamous neoplasia of the uterine cervix. There is a parallel association with HPV, with some blot hybridization studies detecting at least 1,000 viral copies/cell in all patients. Viral DNA of HPV, particularly serotype 16, has been demonstrated in more than half of invasive carcinomas. The resulting spectrum of preneoplastic and neoplastic changes includes VaIN I, II, and III, microinvasive, and invasive carcinomas. These lesions may be multifocal. Intraepithelial lesions (VaIN) are rare in the vagina, compared to those involving the cervix or vulva, with an annual incidence of only 0.3/100,000 women. In as many as 66–80% of cases, there is prior or synchronous preinvasive or invasive squamous neoplasia elsewhere in the genital tract. Vaginal cancer can spread through direct extension to the adjacent pelvic organs, soft tissue, or pelvic bones. Lymphatic dissemination results in involvement of pelvic and paraaortic lymph nodes; lower vaginal tumors spread to the inguinal-femoral lymph nodes. Hematogenous dissemination affects distant organs, particularly lung, liver, and bone.

Specimen Handling

The treatment of primary vaginal carcinoma and the specimens submitted for consultation vary with the location and stage of the tumor. For stage I lesions involving the upper third of the vagina, surgical treatment consists of radical hysterectomy, upper vaginectomy, and pelvic lymph-node dissection (Fig. 3.1). For lesions involving the lower third, radical vulvovaginectomy and bilateral inguinal lymph-node dissection are performed. Determination of extension of the tumor to the subvaginal tissue (stage II), to the pelvic wall (stage III), or beyond the true pelvis (stage IV) is essential, since tumor stage is the most important prognostic factor. Advanced cases respond to radiation, therefore ultraradical surgery or exenteration with removal of the bladder and/or rectum is not usually considered unless the tumor fails to respond adequately to radiation.

Gross examination of the tumor, its dimensions, its relationship to any attached organs, and the distance to the surgical margins should be noted and sampled along the narrowest point. The exposed soft tissues that surround the uterus and vagina are inked. The lower margins of resection can be submitted for frozen section evaluation. In cases where the bladder or rectum is included in the resection (anterior or posterior exenteration respectively), additional margins to be evaluated include urethral, ureteral, proximal, and distal rectal margins.

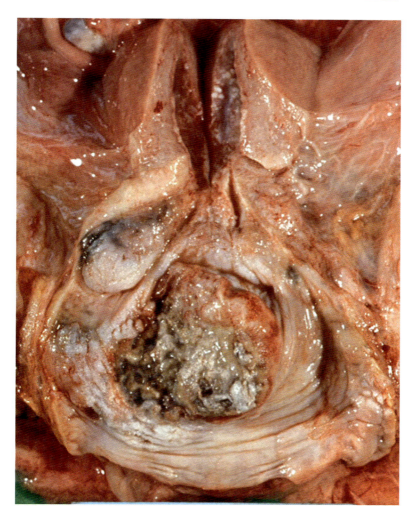

FIGURE 3.1 Radical vaginectomy for squamous cell carcinoma. The fungating vaginal tumor involves the upper two thirds of the vagina, but spares the cervix and is separated from the vulva by a wide margin of normal vagina. There is extensive surface ulceration and necrosis.

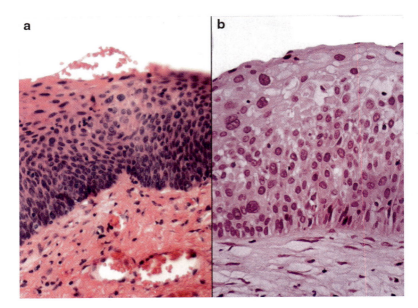

FIGURE 3.2 Vaginal intraepithelial neoplasia. (a) A high grade lesion (VaIN III) with cellular crowding, high N/C ratio, hyperchromasia and nuclear pleomorphism involving almost the entire thickness of the epithelium. (b) A biopsy from a vaginal lesion (VaIN II) that developed 6 years after radiotherapy for cervical cancer. The nuclear atypia and cellular crowding is less than that in Fig. 3.2a, and involves about half the thickness of the epithelium (H&E, medium power).

Interpretation

Frozen sections play a limited role in the diagnosis of VaIN lesions. They are not optimal for accurate grading of early neoplastic lesions in view of the freezing artifact inherent in the technique. Such examination, however, is helpful in excluding the presence of stromal invasion in suspicious areas (Fig. 3.2). If the lesion is limited to the vagina, it can be treated by laser, 5-FU, or partial vaginectomy. Vaginal intraepithelial neoplasia may be also encountered following or in association with cervical squamous epithelial neoplasia (Fig. 3.3).

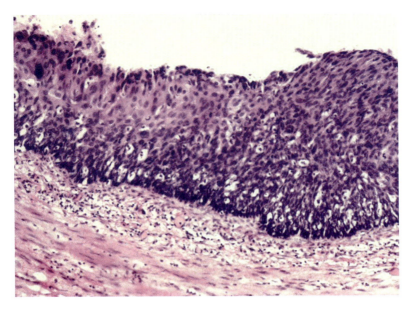

FIGURE 3.3 Vaginal intraepithelial neoplasia. This lesion was encountered partially lining an inclusion cyst. There is complete involvement of the entire thickness of the epithelium by a high-grade intraepithelial neoplastic change. The patient had a history of cervical cancer (H&E, medium power).

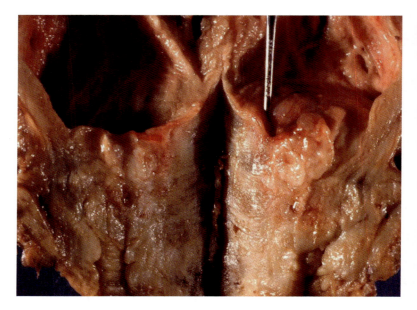

FIGURE 3.4 Radical vaginectomy for squamous cell carcinoma. This vaginal tumor developed 15 years following radiation therapy for squamous cell carcinoma of the cervix. The tumor infiltrated the bladder anteriorly and showed extensive sclerosis.

Invasive squamous cell carcinoma arises more commonly in the upper third of the vagina. It can appear as a polypoid, ulcerating, or flat lesion (Figs. 3.4 and 3.5). Nests of keratinizing or nonkeratinizing malignant cells, similar to those encountered in the cervix, infiltrate subepithelial tissues (Fig. 3.6). Since small superficially invasive vaginal cancers can still have poor outcome, the term microinvasive carcinoma has not been accepted.

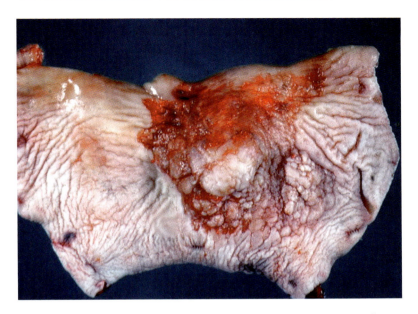

FIGURE 3.5 Squamous cell carcinoma. The vaginectomy specimen shows a fungating mass with surface ulceration and hemorrhage. From Ramzy I. Essentials of gynecologic and obstetric pathology. Norwalk: Appleton Century Crofts; 1983. p. 77. Used with permission.

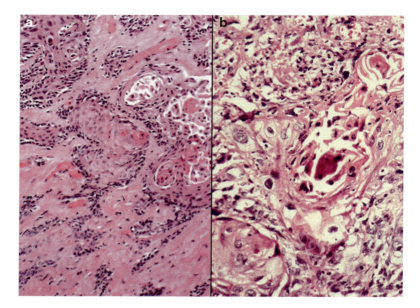

FIGURE 3.6 Invasive squamous cell carcinoma. (a) Nests of squamous cell carcinoma invade the subepithelial tissues. They have irregular shapes and pointed edges. This is a well-differentiated keratinizing tumor (H&E, low power). (b) Squamous cell carcinoma with keratinization, necrosis and focal calcification (H&E, medium power).

In addition to the usual type of squamous cell carcinoma, rare variants can involve the vagina, including verrucous carcinoma, sarcomatoid carcinoma, and lymphoepithelioma-like carcinomas. Verrucous carcinoma poses a challenge in view of the high degree of differentiation and lack of significant atypia, despite its tendency to recur and occasional local aggressive behavior (Figs. 3.7 and 3.8). It has a pushing border that invades deeply as broad bulbous epithelial nests with smooth outlines, unlike the classic squamous carcinoma nests that have pointed projections (refer to Chap. 2).

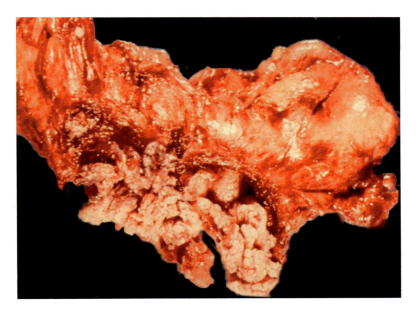

FIGURE 3.7 Verrucous carcinoma. The neoplastic fronds originated from the vagina and infiltrated the rectal wall, resulting in a 3 cm × 2 cm mucosal ulcer (see Fig. 3.8).

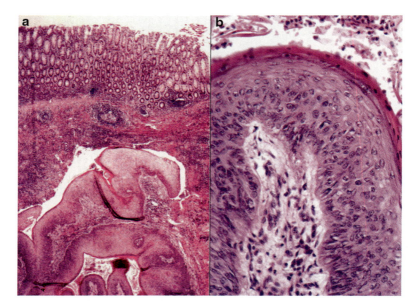

FIGURE 3.8 Verrucous carcinoma. (**a**) Verrucous finger like processes infiltrate the wall of the rectum. The section is from the colon around the ulcerated mucosa (H&E, low power). From Ramzy I, Smout MS, Collins JA. Verrucous carcinoma of the vagina, Amer J Clin Pathol. 1976;65:644–53. (**b**) Despite the aggressive and locally infiltrative nature of the tumor, the papillary fronds are covered by relatively uniform squamous epithelium. They have bulbous pushing, rather than infiltrating, borders (H&E, medium power).

Differential Diagnostic Considerations

Squamous cell carcinoma should be differentiated from other papillary squamous lesions, particularly squamous cell papilloma and condyloma acuminatum.

Squamous cell papillomas are rare in the vagina, compared to condylomas. They lack nuclear atypia or subepithelial nests seen in invasive squamous cell carcinoma. *Condylomata acuminata* involving the vagina can have a papillary or flat-growth pattern. The epithelial cell nuclei are slightly enlarged, but the atypia is only minimal, and the presence of koilocytic changes and multinucleation are helpful features (Fig. 3.9). Any significant atypia reflects an early neoplastic process Condylomata may also show significant atypia as a result of local treatment, but the chromatin in such cases is smudged and mitotic activity is lacking. *Postradiation epithelial*

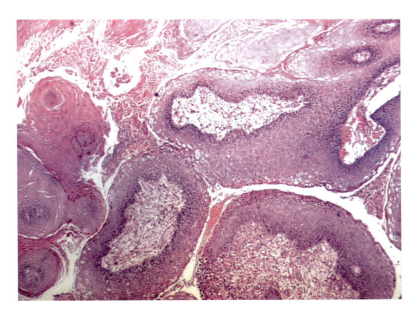

FIGURE 3.9 Condyloma acuminatum. Finger like processes showing hyperkeratosis, parakeratosis, focal koilocytosis, but lacking significant nuclear atypia. If atypia is evident, it should be reported. However, such an evaluation is rarely requested intraoperatively, since it does not influence the immediate management and the clinical history is usually helpful (H&E, low power).

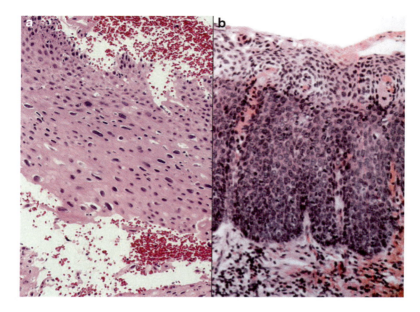

FIGURE 3.10 Postradiation changes. (a) Mild nuclear atypia without increase in N/C ratio (H&E, medium power). (b) Postradiation dysplasia (VaIN III) showing increased N/C ratio with enlarged hyperchromatic nuclei, involving most of the thickness of the epithelium. This change may develop even after 20 years of exposure to radiation, and may be associated with development of primary invasive carcinoma of the vagina (H&E, medium power).

atypia may develop in patients following treatment for cervical cancer, and should be differentiated from VaIN. Although the nuclei of irradiated cells are enlarged and hyperchromatic, they have smudged degenerated chromatin and are associated with cytomegaly, thus the N/C ratio is not increased. However, true VaIN as well as invasive carcinoma may subsequently develop many years after radiotherapy for cervical cancer (Fig. 3.10).

VAGINECTOMY FOR ADENOCARCINOMA

Clinical Background and Specimen Handling

Vaginal adenocarcinomas, including the clear cell variant, are uncommon malignancies. In most cases, adenocarcinomas represent tumor extension from the cervix or endometrium, and such a possibility should be excluded prior to concluding that the tumor has originated from the vagina. Management of vaginal adenocar-

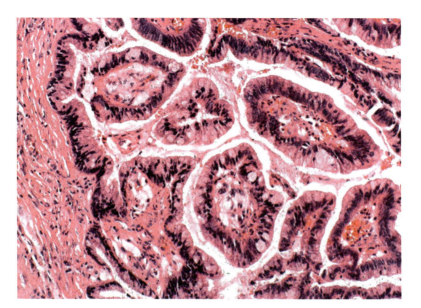

FIGURE 3.11 Adenocarcinoma. The primary adenocarcinoma was not associated with other neoplasms of the cervix or other organs. The columnar epithelium shows stratification (H&E medium power).

cinoma is usually along the same lines of those for squamous cell carcinoma, and the resulting specimens submitted for consultation are generally handled in a similar fashion. Of the various types of adenocarcinoma, clear cell carcinoma tends to be associated with high incidence of lymph-node metastases, approximately 16% in stage I and 30% or more in stage II (DiSaia 2007).

Interpretation
Vaginal adenocarcinoma may show endometrioid, mucinous, papillary serous, clear-cell, or small-cell morphology (Fig. 3.11). The carcinoma may also be associated with endometriosis, adenosis, mesonephric duct remnants, or neuroendocrine cells. Definitive classification is often difficult on frozen section. Vaginal endometri-

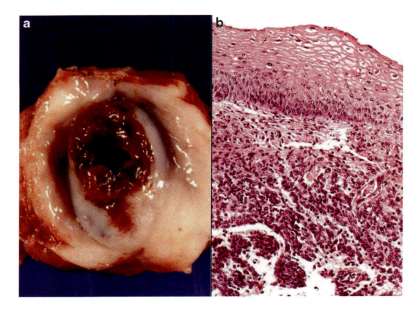

FIGURE 3.12 Endometriosis. (a) The cervix shows areas of hemorrhagic endometriotic tissue around the os. The vagina has minute foci of *bluish areas* (*arrows*) indicative of endometriosis (H&E, medium power). (b) The subepithelial tissues of the vagina show endometrial stroma and some disrupted degenerated glands. Nuclear enlargement may be encountered but such nuclei show homogenized chromatin, evidence of degeneration (H&E, medium power).

osis can be identified in many of the primary vaginal *endometrioid adenocarcinomas* and is important in indicating a primary vaginal tumor, rather than a secondary spread from the endometrium (Fig. 3.12).

Clear cell carcinoma involves the anterior wall of the upper vagina and is often associated with adenosis. The neoplasm may be large polypoid, flat, or ulcerated. The tumor cells have a clear cytoplasm, and form glands or line spaces in a hobnail fashion, similar to those encountered in the endometrium and ovary (Fig. 3.13) (see also Chaps. 5 and 6).

Neuroendocrine carcinomas can be encountered in the vagina. Similar to other malignancies, careful search for a primary elsewhere should be performed before concluding that the vagina is the pri-

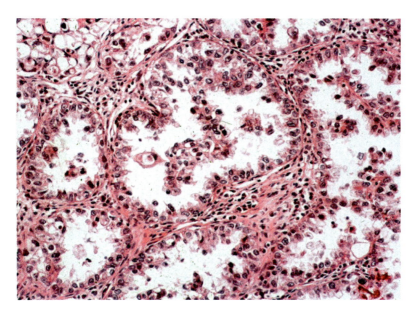

FIGURE 3.13 Clear cell adenocarcinoma. Glandular cleftlike spaces of variable shapes, mostly lined by single layer of cells arranged in hobnail pattern. The nuclei are pleomorphic and the cytoplasm varies from eosinophilic to clear. A papillary pattern is seen in some areas. The irregularly shaped glands are separated by edematous or loose stroma. Other areas (not illustrated) may show solid nests of neoplastic cells (H&E, medium power).

mary source. The neoplasm shows the usual nuclear and cytoplasmic features of neuroendocrine tumors, although proper classification beyond a poorly differentiated carcinoma may not be feasible at the time of intraoperative consultation. Immunohistochemistry is usually needed to confirm the neuroendocrine nature of the tumor (Figs. 3.14 and 3.15).

Differential Diagnostic Considerations

Several benign lesions can mimic adenocarcinomas. These include adenosis, prolapse of fallopian tube, microglandular hyperplasia, endometriosis, and Arias-Stella reaction as well as some cysts. A detailed description of these lesions is beyond the scope of this text, but, in general, they have circumscribed borders and

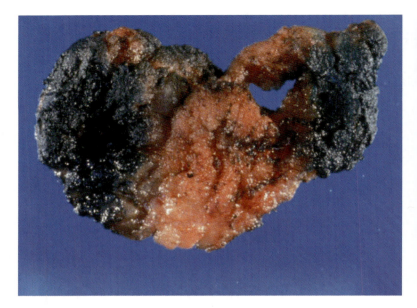

FIGURE 3.14 Neuroendocrine carcinoma. The tumor resulted in irregular thickening of the vaginal wall and focal ulceration. Differentiation from other types of malignancies require histologic examination of the neoplasm.

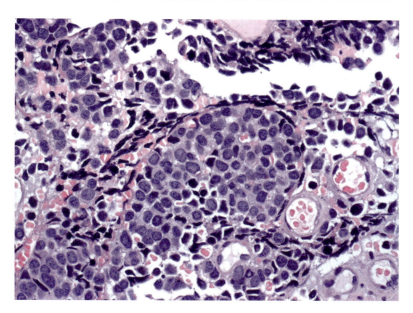

FIGURE 3.15 Neuroendocrine carcinoma. Solid nests and cords of highly malignant cells infiltrate the subepithelial tissues. The large nuclei show pleomorphism and coarsely granular salt-and-pepper chromatin pattern. A rare cell cluster shows cytoplasmic vacuolization suggesting a glandular differentiation. The neoplastic cells stain strongly for neuroendocrine immunohistochemical markers (H&E, high power).

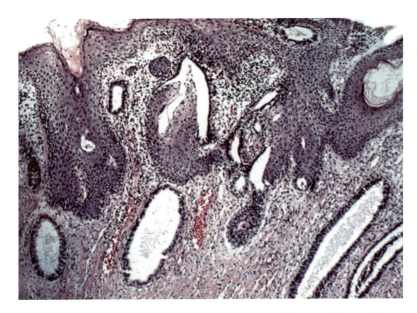

FIGURE 3.16 Adenosis. The vaginal squamous epithelium and the subepithelial tissues show clefts and glands lined by Müllerian epithelium (H&E, low power). Image used as a courtesy of Dr. William A. Meriwether, San Antonio, Texas.

exhibit only minimal cytologic atypia. Adenosis is usually seen in the upper vagina in approximately a third of patients who were exposed in utero to diethylstilbestrol (DES) (Fig. 3.16). The glandular epithelium replaces the native squamous epithelium and consists of glands lined by mucinous, serous, or endometrial-type epithelial cells, often associated with squamous metaplasia. Unfortunately, freezing limits the ability to ascertain detailed nuclear features in some cases and subsequently causes diagnostic difficulty. Prolapse of the fallopian tube appears as a granular area in the vaginal vault several months after vaginal hysterectomy. If the original hysterectomy was performed for an endometrial adenocarcinoma, the presence of these areas may raise the suspicion of a local recurrence. The fronds form distorted glandular spaces, but unlike adenocarcinoma, there is intense inflammation and granulation-like tissue (Fig. 3.17). Microglandular hyperplasia and Arias-Stella changes are rarely encountered in the vagina; the hyperchromatic nuclei in both conditions manifest degenerative smudged chromatin that contrasts with the crisp chromatin in true malignant cells (refer to Chap. 4

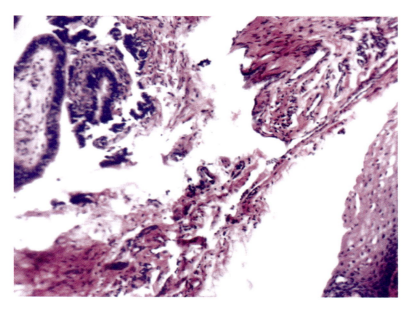

FIGURE 3.17 Prolapsed fallopian tube. The upper part of the vagina in this patient showed an area of granulation 7 weeks after hysterectomy for endometrial adenocarcinoma. The mucosal folds are of tubal epithelium that shows no evidence of cell stratification or nuclear pleomorphism. There is usually intense inflammatory response in subepithelial tissues (H&E, low power).

for more detailed discussion). Vaginal cysts or vestigial remnants may be encountered in the wall of the vagina. These are lined by a single layer of cuboidal or Müllerian epithelium, with no cellular crowding or nuclear atypia.

VAGINECTOMY FOR SARCOMAS AND OTHER SPINDLE CELL LESIONS

Clinical Background

Sarcomas, malignant mixed Müllerian tumors, aggressive angiomyxomas as well as leiomyomas, angiomyofibroblastomas, and benign rhabdomyomas are among the spindle cell neoplasms reported in the vagina. Except for leiomyoma, the most common mesenchymal tumor, these are only rarely encountered. The diagnosis in most of these cases is established by prior biopsies; the role of frozen section is usually limited to evaluation of resection margins in malignant tumors. The vaginectomy specimens are handled as

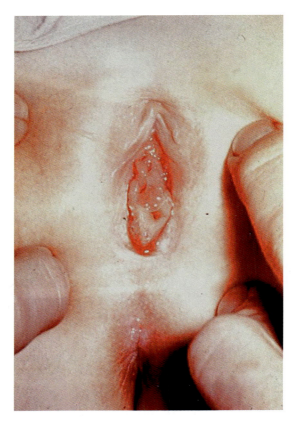

FIGURE 3.18 Rhabdomyosarcoma. Grape like polypoid tumor is filling the vagina and protruding from the introitus of a 5-year-old child (Courtesy of Dr. Carl J. Pauerstein, San Antonio, Texas).

previously described under squamous cell carcinoma. It is imperative that material from the original biopsy, if available, be reviewed prior to evaluating the specimen from the definitive surgery by frozen section. This allows comparing the two specimens and differentiating low-grade lesions from reactive stromal changes.

Interpretation and Differential Diagnostic Considerations

Embryonal rhabdomyosarcoma (sarcoma botryoides) is the most common malignant tumor of the vagina in infants, mostly affecting children younger than 5 years. The soft bulky grapelike polypoid tumor may fill the vagina (Fig. 3.18). The edematous core contains primi-

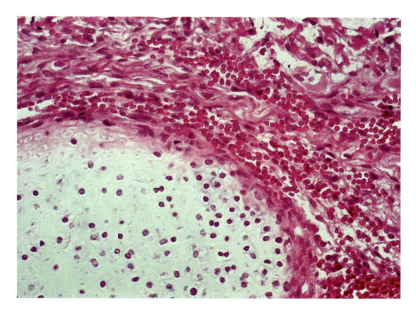

FIGURE 3.19 Rhabdomyosarcoma. This tumor was resected from the upper vagina in a 19-year-old patient. Mesenchymal tissues including cartilage, smooth muscle and vascular tissues are among the components identified in this neoplasm (H&E, medium power).

tive small mesenchymal cells with several mitotic figures, as well as elongated or strap-like rhabdomyoblasts showing cross striations. A zone of densely arranged small undifferentiated mesenchymal cells is seen under the surface epithelium (cambium layer), and an occasional island of cartilage may be present (Figs. 3.19 and 3.20). Immunoreactivity for myoD1, myogenin and desmin confirms the diagnosis. *Leiomyosarcoma* may be encountered in the vagina, and its characteristics as well as features that help differentiating it from leiomyoma are detailed in Chap. 5.

The differential diagnosis of vaginal sarcomas encompasses several benign conditions were marked cytologic atypia may result in a false positive diagnosis, particularly when freezing artifact hinders accurate evaluation of nuclear and cytoplasmic features.

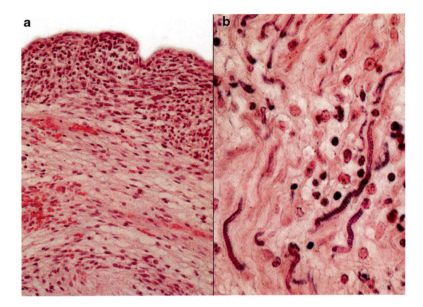

FIGURE 3.20 Rhabdomyosarcoma (same case as Fig. 3.19). (**a**) The edematous polypoid structures consist of loose mesenchymal tissue with a dense subepithelial layer of primitive cells (cambium layer). (**b**) Elongated fibers of rhabdomyoblasts are seen among other primitive mesenchymal loose tissue (H&E, medium power).

Generous sampling of the suspected areas and the use of special and immunostains may be necessary to evaluate such specimens. Table 3.1 lists the common differential diagnostic problems in vaginal intraoperative consultations for sarcomas.

Reactive changes, including those that follow radiation therapy for cervical carcinoma, granulation tissue, and posthysterectomy spindle cell nodules can be a source of difficulties. Such vaginal biopsies should not be submitted for frozen section evaluation, particularly since they rarely influence immediate management decisions. *Fibroepithelial polyps* (myofibroblastomas) form solitary or multiple papillary masses in the lower part of the vagina. The papillae have edematous cores covered by squamous epithelium

TABLE 3.1 Differential diagnostic considerations in vaginal malignancies.

Squamous cell carcinoma	Adenocarcinoma	Sarcoma
Papilloma	Adenosis	Reactive stroma
Condyloma acuminatum	Tubal prolapse	Radiation
Radiation	Microglandular hyperplasia	Spindle cell nodule
Fibroepithelial polyp		Granulation tissue
		Fibroepithelial polyp

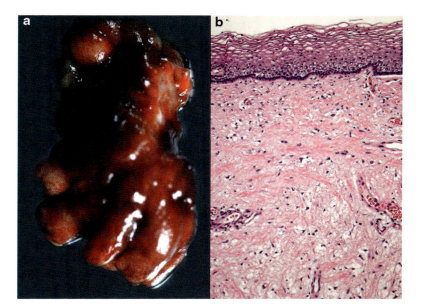

FIGURE 3.21 Fibroepithelial polyp. (**a**) The polypoid mass was resected from the vagina of a 55 years old patient. There is evidence of hemorrhage, probably as a result of partial torsion (H&E, low power). (**b**) The polyp has an edematous stroma and is covered by uniform squamous epithelium (H&E, low power).

with bland nuclei. The stroma may be cellular and consists of polygonal or elongated cells with pointed cytoplasmic processes, and multinucleation is not uncommon (Figs. 3.21 and 3.22). The tumor may show mild cytologic stromal atypia, but the patient's

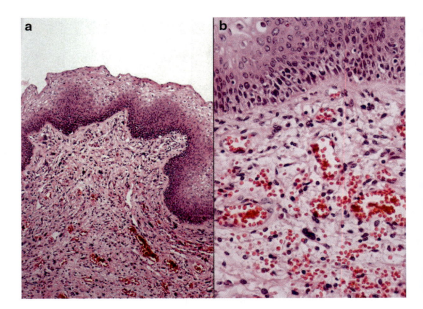

FIGURE 3.22 Fibroepithelial polyp, postpartum. (**a**) The stratified squamous epithelium covers a stroma of spindle cells with focal nuclear pleomorphism (H&E, low power). (**b**) Higher power showing the nuclear atypia of the stromal cells (H&E, medium power).

age, association with pregnancy or hormonal therapy, and the lack of epithelial atypia, strap-cell or dense stroma differentiate fibroepithelial polyps from rhabdomyosarcoma. *Aggressive angiomyxoma* is often a bulky mass, with thick-walled blood vessels and only rare multinucleated cells, unlike fibroepithelial polyps. The tumor also lacks the small undifferentiated mesenchymal cells and the rhabdomyoblasts that characterize embryonal rhabdomyosarcoma (Fig. 3.23).

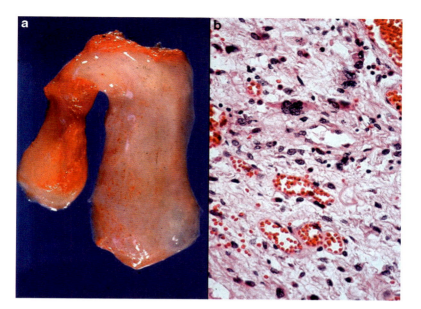

FIGURE 3.23 Aggressive angiomyxoma. (**a**) An edematous polypoid mass resected from the upper vagina of a 35-year-old patient. The age is helpful in differentiating this from rhabdomyosarcoma. (**b**) Myxoid and vascular stroma, showing nuclear pleomorphism (H&E, medium power).

RECOMMENDED READING

Balamurugan A, Ahmed F, Saraiya M, et al. Potential role of human papillomavirus in the development of subsequent primary in situ and invasive cancers among cervical cancer survivors. Cancer. 2008;113:2919–25.

Bigby SM, Symmans PJ, Miller MV, et al. Aggressive angiomyxoma of the female genital tract and pelvis- Clinicopathologic features with immunohistochemical analysis. Internat J Gynecol Pathol. 2011;30:505–13.

Boonlikit S, Noinual N. Vaginal intraepithelial neoplasia: a retrospective analysis of clinical features and colpohistology. J Obstet Gynecol Res. 2010;36:94–100.

Creasman WT, Phillips JL, Menck HR. The National Cancer Data Base report on cancer of vagina. Cancer. 1998;83:1033–40.

Diakomanolis E, Stefanidis K, Rodolakis A, et al. Vaginal intraepithelial neoplasia a report of 102 cases. Eu J Gynaecol Oncol. 2002;23:547–9.

DiSaia PJ, Creasman WT. Clinical gynecologic oncology. 7th ed. Philadelphia, PA: Mosby-Elsevier; 2007.

Dunn LJ, Napier JG. Primary carcinoma of the vagina. Am J Obstet Gynecol. 1966;96:1112.

Ferreira M, Crespo M, Martins L, Felix A. HPV DNA detection and genotyping in 21 cases of primary invasive squamous cell carcinoma of vagina. Mod pathol. 2008;21:968–72.

Frank SJ, Deavers MT, Jhingran A, et al. Primary adenocarcinoma of the vagina not associated with diethylstilbestrol (DES) exposure. Gynecol Oncol. 2007;105:470–4.

Gallum DG, Talledo OE, Shah KJ, Hayes C. Invasive squamous cell carcinoma of the vagina: a 14 year study. Obstet Gynecol. 1987;69:782.

Hellman K, Lundell M, Silfversward C, et al. Clinical and histopathologic factors related to prognosis in primary squamous cell carcinoma of the vagina. Int J Gynecol Cancer. 2006;16:1201–11.

Hellmann K, Silfversward C, Nilsson B, et al. Primary carcinoma of the vagina: factors influencing the age at diagnosis. The radiumhemmet series 1956–96. Int J Gynecol Cancer. 2004;14:491–501.

Lilic V, Filipovic S, Visnjic M, Zivadinovic R. Primary carcinoma of vagina. J BUON. 2010;15:241–7.

Rome RM, England PG. Management of vaginal intraepithelial neoplasia: a series of 132 cases with long term follow-up. Int J Gynecol Cancer. 2000;10:382–90.

Sinha B, Stehman F, Schilder J, et al. Indiana University experience in the management of vaginal cancer. Int J Gynecol Cancer. 2009;19:686–93.

Staats PN, Clements PB, Young RH. Primary endometrioid adenocarcinoma of the vagina: a clinicopathologic study of 18 cases. Am J Surg Pathol. 2007;31:1490–501.

Van Dam P, Sonnemans H, van Dam PJ, et al. Sentinel node detection in patients with vaginal carcinoma. Gynecol Oncol. 2004;92:89–92.

Verloop J, Rookus MA, van Leeuwen FE. Prevalence of gynecologic cancer in women exposed to diethylstilbestrol in utero. N Engl J Med. 2000;342:1838.

Weinstock MA. Malignant melanoma of the vulva and vagina in the United States: patterns of incidence and population-based estimates of survival. Am J Obstet Gynecol. 1994;171:1225.

Chapter 4
Uterine Cervix

Intraoperative consultation is often sought for specimens from the cervix. Almost all consultations are related to cervical carcinoma, the sixth most common solid malignancy among women in the United States. Some specimens are submitted for gross consultation only, but the majority requires frozen section examination to assess the presence and extent of malignancy (Table 4.1). In approximately 70% of patients with cervical cancer, the disease is limited to the cervix. The diagnosis is initially established usually by a punch biopsy. Patients with pre-invasive disease (FIGO Stage 0) and patients with superficial invasion (FIGO Stage IA) who desire to preserve fertility can be treated with limited procedures, including loop electrosurgical excision procedure (LEEP) excision and conization. Some modalities, such as cryosurgery and laser vaporization, destroy the tissue, and no samples are submitted for intraoperative consultation by frozen section. Advanced stages of malignancies require more extensive surgical resections to include, in addition to the cervix, the uterine body, and often both tubes and ovaries, while others are treated with radiation and/or chemotherapy.

The different types of specimens received for consultation will be considered first, followed by discussion of the individual lesions and the different diagnostic issues encountered in each of these conditions.

CERVICAL PUNCH BIOPSY

This common diagnostic office procedure is often performed under colposcopic guidance and specimens are rarely submitted for intraoperative consultation. If a biopsy is submitted, the pathologist should resist the temptation to freeze the sample in order to satisfy

TABLE 4.1 Reasons for intraoperative consultations in the cervix.

- Presence of malignancy
- Type of carcinoma
- Depth of invasion by carcinoma
- Extent of invasion by carcinoma
- Adequacy of resection at surgical margins (exocervix, endocervix and soft tissue)

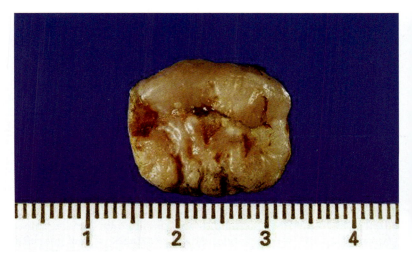

FIGURE 4.1 LEEP specimen: This specimen, obtained as an office procedure by a loop electrosurgical excision, illustrates an irregular surface and includes the entire circumference of the transformation zone.

the curiosity of the surgeon. Freezing the artifact may prohibit establishing a definitive diagnosis on permanent sections; small lesions can be destroyed while attempting to "face" the block, and the assessment of margins in such small, poorly oriented specimens is not reliable. In almost all circumstances, the patient's interest is better served by examining a properly fixed paraffin-embedded tissue sample.

LOOP ELECTROSURGICAL EXCISION PROCEDURE

This procedure allows the resection of the transformation zone (TZ) and nearby abnormal tissue, following the delineation of the entire lesion by colposcopy (Fig. 4.1). Many specimens are accompanied by a "top hat," a separate excision of the endocervical margin at the top of the original LEEP, to ensure a clear endocervical margin. Since LEEP excisions are usually performed in an office setting, they are unlikely to be submitted for frozen sections. If a consultation is indicated, the transformation zone and top hat specimens are treated in a similar manner to the cervical cone described below.

CERVICAL CONE BIOPSY

Clinical Background

Cervical conization plays an important role in the definitive treatment of high-grade squamous intraepithelial lesions or microinvasive cervical carcinomas. Its use, strictly for diagnostic purposes, has been greatly replaced by performing punch biopsies under colposcopic guidance. The procedure implies a conical excision of the cervical transformation zone and canal, performed with laser or surgical blade (cold knife excision). The height and size of the cone vary with the perceived extent of the lesion (Fig. 4.2).

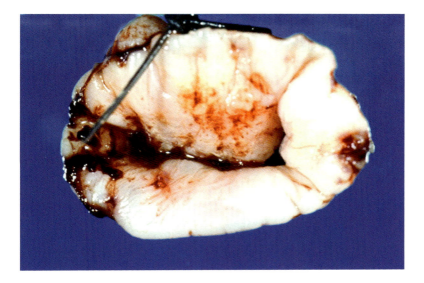

FIGURE 4.2 Cone biopsy: A suture marks the 12 o'clock position. In view of the *transverse shape* of the external os in parous patients, preparing well oriented *perpendicular* slices of the cone at the 3 and 9 o'clock positions may be difficult, and result in incomplete sections that may not include the transformation zone.

Specimen Handling

By convention, the ectocervix is described as a clock face with the most superior midpoint of the anterior lip designated as 12 o'clock. This point is usually oriented by the surgeon using a suture. After orientation of the specimen in the laboratory, the lateral and endocervical mucosal margins are inked using different colors, and the specimen opened along the 12 o'clock line. Sections are submitted and designated as to their clock-face orientation and should include the squamocolumnar junction (Fig. 4.3). Irregularly shaped cone biopsies, as often is the case in parous women, are sometimes difficult to cut at the 3 and 9 o'clock positions, and these sections might only include muscle and soft tissues without any mucosa.

Interpretation

Evaluation by frozen sections should be limited to those cases where the immediate operative management depends on the findings, such as in patients with in situ carcinoma, microinvasive carcinoma or extensive high grade dysplasia who will undergo simple hysterectomy after biopsy. Frozen section examination of the cone biopsy is performed to determine the extent of the disease, to exclude the presence of deep invasion, and to assess the involvement of endocervical or lateral-deep margins of excision. The degree of accuracy of the procedure enables the surgeon to make an immediate decision about definitive therapy. Furthermore, frozen section of conization specimens followed by immediate hysterectomy offers the advantage of a single procedure, thereby reducing the risk of additional anesthesia and decreasing patients' expenses. Evaluation of the degree of dysplasia by frozen sections is not recommended since freezing artifacts may hinder the assessment of nuclear sizes and crowding (Figs. 4.4–4.6) and results in a higher degree (up to 27%) of discrepancy with permanent sections (Woodford 1986). Such discrepancy may lead to unnecessary hysterectomies in patients for whom the frozen section shows a more severe lesion than is found on permanent sections.

It is important to correlate frozen section interpretation with the patient's previous diagnostic biopsy. In cases where findings are discordant, it is advisable to delay treatment until permanent sections can be evaluated.

Limitations of Conization

Although freezing cone biopsies is accurate in detecting invasive disease, the procedure has its limitations. Numerous blocks and slides are prepared for each case, and a considerable amount of

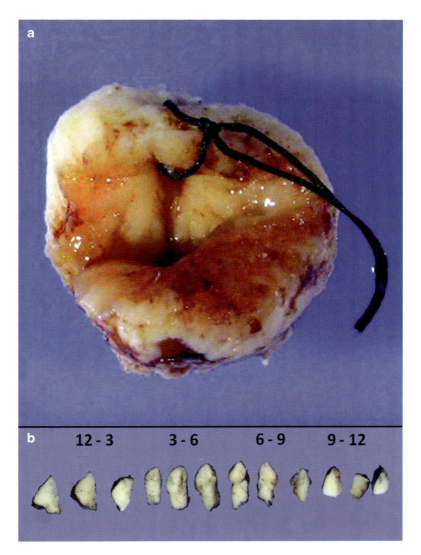

FIGURE 4.3 Cone biopsy: (**a**) The outer surface of cervical cone biopsy, including the endocervical top, is inked prior to opening at 12 o' clock position. (**b**) Proper cutting, labeling and orientation of the slices is critical in minimizing the risk of misinterpreting invasion and involvement of the margin.

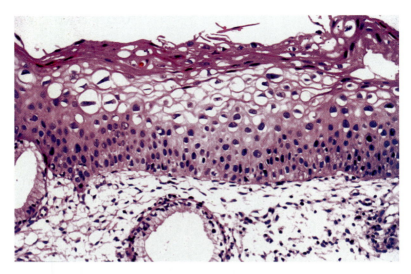

FIGURE 4.4 Artifactual vacuoles versus HPV: Frozen sections can present difficulty in differentiating HPV from artifactual vacuolization due to freezing artifact. The latter affects the epithelium in a diffuse pattern, while involvement of isolated cells, multinucleation and presence of nuclear atypia support the diagnosis of HPV (H&E, medium power).

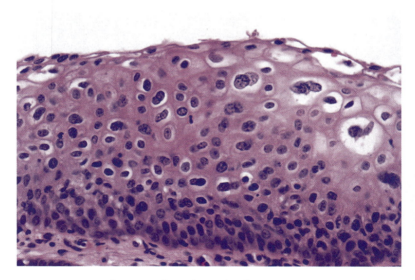

FIGURE 4.5 HPV changes with moderate dysplasia (CIN II). Multinucleation, koilocytosis with increasingly bizarre nuclei closer to the surface are features of HPV. The cellular crowding and atypia involving about half the thickness of the epithelium indicate moderate dysplasia (H&E, high power).

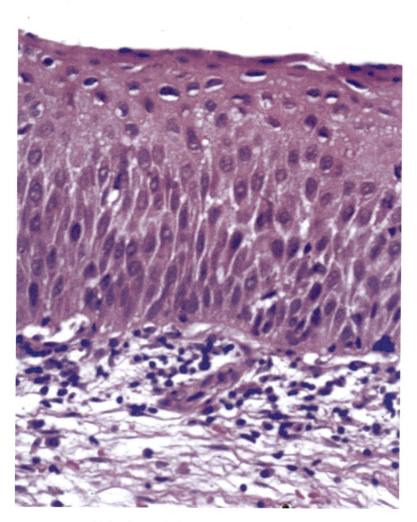

FIGURE 4.6 Mild dysplasia. Slight nuclear crowding and hyperchromasia is mostly limited to the lower third of the epithelium. The surface epithelial cells show normal orientation (H&E, medium power).

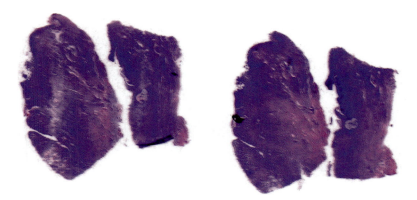

FIGURE 4.7 Embedding two cervical slices of the cone per block cuts the time required for cutting and staining. However, it requires uniform thickness of the two slices to avoid losing tissue by having to face one slice more than the other.

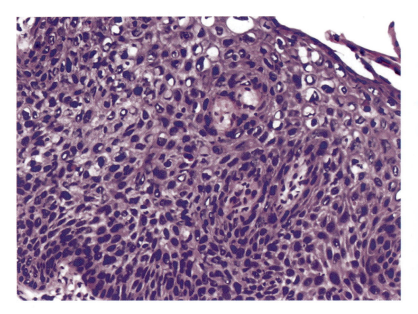

FIGURE 4.8 CIN III and proper orientation. Tangential cuts, as evidenced by the presence of small islands of stroma, may interfere with proper assessment of the thickness and extent of involvement of the epithelium by intraepithelial neoplasia (H&E, medium power).

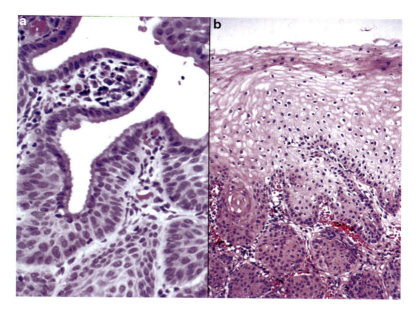

FIGURE 4.9 Squamous metaplasia. (**a**) In early phases, uniform bland hyperplastic reserve cells maintain a surface layer of columnar cells (H&E, medium power). From Ramzy I. Essentials of gynecologic and obstetric pathology. Norwalk: Appleton Century Crofts; 1983. p. 96. Used with permission. (**b**) More mature metaplasia loses the columnar epithelium. The nests of epithelial cells are close to the surface, well defined, with a smooth outer margin (H&E, low power).

time is involved while the patient is on the operating room table. One way of speeding up the process is to put two pieces of tissue in each block, thus cutting the number of slides and time of evaluation roughly by 50% (Fig. 4.7). Such a technique, however, carries the risk of losing a focal lesion in one piece while trying to face the block to expose the second piece. Proper orientation is critical in assessing the thickness of the epithelium involved by dysplasia (Fig. 4.8). It is also important not to misinterpret the islands of squamous metaplasia in the superficial stroma as evidence of stromal invasion. These islands, even when sectioned tangentially, are well defined, have a smooth border, and are located close to glands and the surface epithelium. They consist of cytologically bland cells with uniform nuclei that are similar to those of the neighboring normal squamous epithelium (Figs. 4.9 and 4.10). Another limitation is

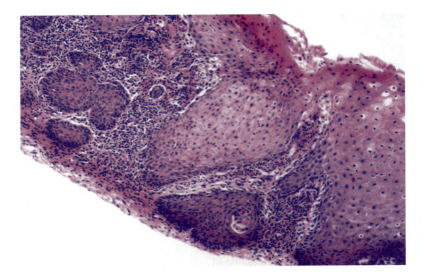

FIGURE 4.10 Pseudoinvasion in CIN III. Tangential cuts may result in islands of squamous epithelium that are separate from the surface epithelium and the glands. However, these are always close to the surface, do not go beyond the level of the glands and additional cuts may show their connection to the surface. Their smooth outer contours and similar morphology of the cells in these islands to those of surface epithelium are helpful differentiating features. Compare to Fig. 4.16 (H&E, low power).

when conization is used to treat carcinoma in situ in young patients who desire to preserve fertility by sparing the uterus. In such cases, evaluation of the endocervical margin at the top of the cone becomes critical. Unfortunately, the diathermy artifactual changes at this area can interfere with this essential evaluation (Fig. 4.11). Complete replacement of the columnar epithelium in a gland by high grade SIL results in rounded nests of neoplastic squamous cells within the cervical stroma. Unlike invasive lesions, these nests have smooth borders because they are contained by basement membrane, are close to the surface, and do not reach deeper than the neighboring native glands (Fig. 4.12). Despite these limitations, the frozen section evaluation of cone biopsies can be used to accurately determine the presence of invasive carcinoma, depth of invasion, and status of endocervical margin, enabling the surgeon to make an immediate decision about definitive therapy.

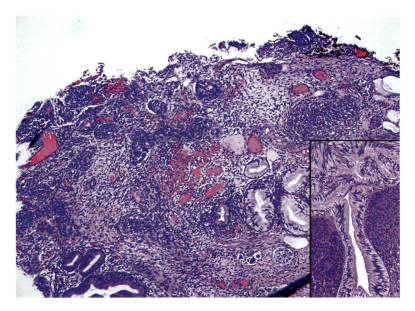

FIGURE 4.11 Effects of diathermy. The epithelium at the endocervical margin shows marked distortion and artifactual changes due to diathermy in two areas. Evaluation of such areas can be extremely difficult since cell architecture and morphology are obliterated. Although recuts may clarify the issue, revision of the resection to obtain a new margin may be necessary to avoid leaving residual neoplastic disease (H&E, low power). Inset illustrates alteration of nuclear morphology and shape of endocervical cells, becoming more spindle-shaped.

Impact of Conization on Management

Simple hysterectomy is performed, after conization, in patients with carcinoma in situ who no longer want to conceive, and in patients with microinvasive carcinoma. The depth of invasion should be measured from the basal lamina of the surface epithelium, or from the overlying endocervical glands involved by HSIL, to the deepest point of invasion. FIGO stage IA1, where the depth of invasion is 3.0 mm or less and the lateral extent is 7.0 mm or less, identifies a group of patients who can be treated without lymphadenectomy or radical hysterectomy. Many gynecologic oncologists feel that the incidence of pelvic lymph node metastasis and tumor recurrence increases when stromal invasion exceeds 3.0 mm. Stage IA2 (invasion greater than 3.0 mm and up to 5.0 mm) and frankly invasive

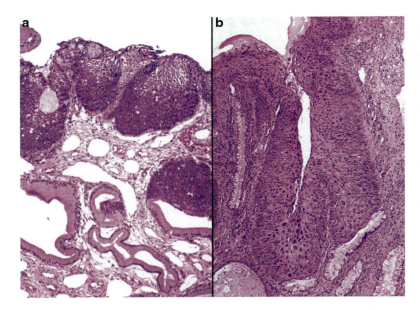

FIGURE 4.12 Endocervical gland involvement by CIN III: (a) and (b) The neoplastic epithelium involves the necks of the glands, but remains closely associated with the columnar epithelium. When the columnar epithelium is completely replaced, leaving only nests of neoplastic squamous cells, the latter maintain their superficial location and are not seen beyond the deepest level of the normal glandular clefts in the vicinity (H&E, low power).

squamous cell carcinomas are treated with radical hysterectomy and pelvic lymph node dissection. Therefore, at the time of frozen section analysis, distinguishing stage IA1 from stages IA2 or beyond is clinically relevant.

RADICAL TRACHELECTOMY

Clinical Background

Radical trachelectomy and laparoscopic pelvic lymphadenectomy are fertility-sparing surgical techniques used as an alternative for radical hysterectomy in early-stage cervical carcinoma. The specific criteria used by gynecologists to select patients for radical trachelectomy include: (1) women with a confirmed diagnosis of squamous, adenosquamous, or adenocarcinoma who wish to preserve fertility; (2) tumors measuring less than 2.0 cm in diameter; (3) FIGO stages

1A1 with lymphovascular invasion, IA2, or IB1; (4) none or minimal endocervical involvement by colposcopy or MRI; and (5) absence of lymph node metastasis at laparoscopy, as confirmed by frozen section of the sentinel or any suspicious node.

Specimen Handling
The procedure can be performed vaginally, preceded by laparoscopic bilateral pelvic lymphadenectomy, or abdominally with pelvic lymphadenectomy. The uterine body is left intact and sutured to the vagina. Radical trachelectomy specimens, therefore, include the cervix, parametria, and a vaginal cuff. Endocervical and endometrial curettages are routinely performed at the time of trachelectomy.

Assessment of Endocervical Margin in Trachelectomy
The status of endocervical margin and the correct assessment of the distance of invasive or in situ carcinoma to this margin is critical for the management of the disease. The entire endocervical margin should be submitted for frozen section examination, preferably using longitudinal sections. The parametria and endocervical/lower uterine margin are inked with different colors. The proximal 1 cm segment is cut off and opened to display its mucosa and examined for presence of tumor. This segment is serially sliced into 10–12 sections, each measuring 3–5 mm, and submitted for frozen section analysis. The remaining cervical tissue is opened longitudinally and examined for residual tumor. Intraoperative assessment of the endocervical margin is crucial since the presence of tumor within 5 mm of that margin necessitates additional resection, including the possibility of complimentary radical hysterectomy. Other margins such as vaginal cuff are submitted for routine paraffin-embedding (Fig. 4.13).

Alternative Techniques of Handling Trachelectomy
Radical trachelectomy specimens can also be handled with a more selective approach. In lesions that are grossly visible, longitudinal sections from the most cephalad portion of the tumor with respect to the endocervical margin are obtained. The final distance to the endocervical margin is considered satisfactory if it is at least 5 mm. It is recommended that more than one sample be submitted. With circumferential lesions, one section per quadrant can be submitted, while in more localized lesions, the number of sections depends on the size of the tumor. Frozen sections can be omitted in grossly normal trachelectomy specimens because 93.3% of these specimens are free of residual invasive disease on permanent sections. However, surgeons must communicate to the pathologist if such cases had

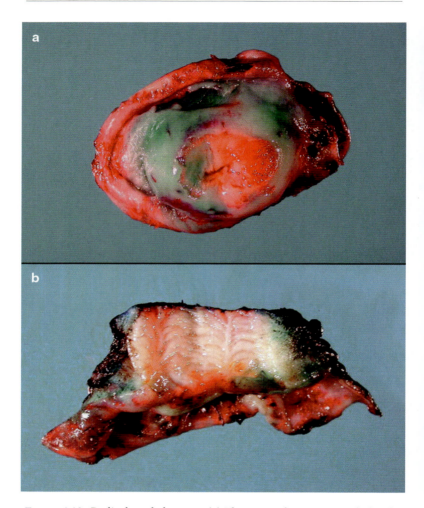

FIGURE 4.13 Radical trachelectomy. (**a**) The resected specimen includes the cervix, paracervical tissues and a vaginal cuff. (**b**) The trachelectomy specimen is opened after the endocervical and parametrial margins are inked. The distance separating neoplastic tissue from the endocervical margin is critical. (**c**) The entire endocervical margin is examined, preferably through longitudinal cuts, as illustrated in this whole mount slide Aperio section (Courtesy Drs. C Diaz Arastia and Claudia Castro).

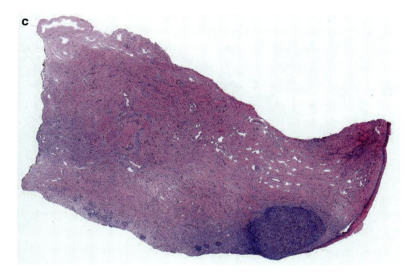

FIGURE 4.13 (continued)

previous LEEP or cone biopsies with positive margins. In such cases, the pathologist may opt to perform frozen section on grossly normal trachelectomy specimens.

TUMORS OF THE CERVIX: EVALUATION AND DIFFERENTIAL DIAGNOSIS

The most common type of cervical malignancies is squamous cell carcinoma, followed by adenocarcinoma and neuroendocrine tumors. Uncommon carcinomas include glassy cell, transitional cell, mesonephric, clear cell, adenoid basal, and adenoid cystic carcinomas. Melanomas, sarcomas, lymphomas, leukemia, and metastatic tumors can also be encountered in the cervix. A detailed discussion of the gross and microscopic features of cervical cancer is beyond the scope of this text, but a concise outline of some aspects of common tumors and different diagnostic issues to be considered within the context of intraoperative consultation is appropriate.

SQUAMOUS CELL CARCINOMA

This is by far the most common histologic type of invasive cervical cancer occurring in about 75–80% of cases. The metaplastic epithelium at the squamocolumnar junction has the greatest propensity for

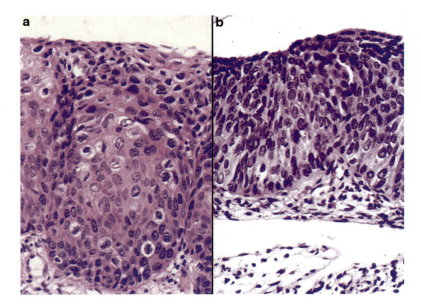

FIGURE 4.14 Cervical intraepithelial neoplasia CIN III. (**a**) There is full thickness involvement by the neoplastic cells, with no attempt at maturation. (**b**) CIN III with a large abnormal vessel running parallel to the surface, consistent with the features reported on colposcopic examination (H&E, medium power). From Ramzy I. Essentials of gynecologic and obstetric pathology. Norwalk: Appleton Century Crofts; 1983. p. 109. Used with permission.

malignant transformation. The association between persistent infection with human papillomavirus and cervical neoplasia has been well documented. High-risk HPV-DNA can be detected in more than 95% of cervical cancer specimens. HPV serotypes 16, 18, 45, 31, and 33 account for 80% of the serotypes found in squamous cell carcinomas.

Squamous neoplasms are classified as intraepithelial, microinvasive, and invasive carcinomas.

Cervical Intraepithelial Neoplasms
These early lesions are often treated conservatively, and issues related to interpretation are considered in detail under conization and trachelectomy. They are illustrated in Figs. 4.14 and 4.15.

Microinvasive Carcinomas
The definition of early invasion (stage IA) endorsed by the Society of Gynecologic Oncologists (SGO), rather than that by International

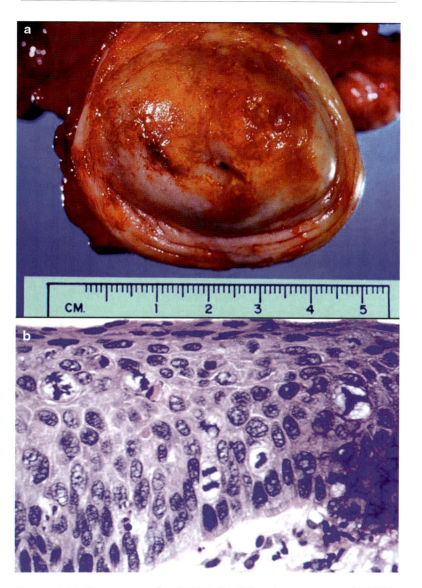

FIGURE 4.15 Hysterectomy for CIN III. (**a**) Although many cases of CIN III lack any significant gross changes, the cervix of this 42 years old patient showed nodular areas that were suspicious for invasive disease. Biopsies, and subsequent extensive histologic examination of the hysterectomy specimen, only revealed an in situ lesion (H&E, high power). (**b**) CIN III with several mitotic figures, some of which are atypical (H&E, high power).

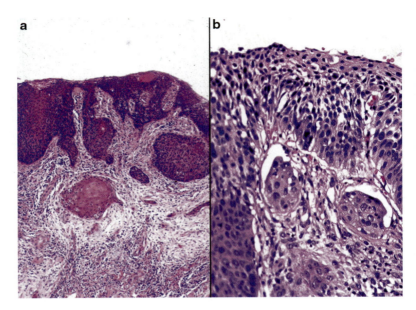

FIGURE 4.16 Microinvasive carcinoma. (**a**) A small nest of malignant squamous epithelium in the superficial stroma. Note the pointed margin of the nest, the eosinophilia of the cytoplasm and the desmoplastic stromal response (H&E, low power). (**b**) Microinvasive carcinoma with two nests invading the superficial stroma. The clear spaces seen partially surrounding the nests are due to shrinkage and should not be interpreted as lymphovascular involvement at the time of frozen section consult; they lack endothelium and only partially surround the tumor tissue. Vascular invasion, however, does not alter the staging (H&E, medium power). From Ramzy I. Essentials of gynecologic and obstetric pathology. Norwalk: Appleton Century Crofts; 1983. p. 129. Used with permission.

Federation of Gynecologists and Obstetricians (FIGO), has now been adopted by many centers. It defines such a tumor as one in which neoplastic cells invade to a depth of 3 mm or less below the base of the epithelium and no more than 7 mm in length, with no capillary lymphatic space involvement (Fig. 4.16). The risk of nodal involvement and recurrence increases with increased depth of invasion. Nodal metastasis of 0.07, 1.9, and 7.8% was reported for lesions invading to the depth of 1 mm or less, 1–2.9, and 3–5 mm, respectively. In some centers, the term "superficially invasive" is preferred, with the notation of depth and width of the lesion, status

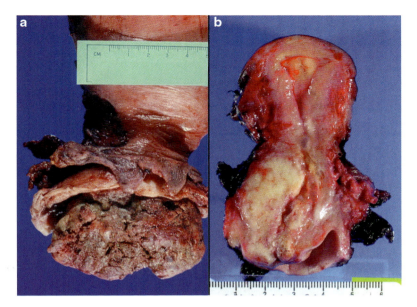

FIGURE 4.17 Invasive squamous cell carcinoma. (**a**) An exophytic tumor protruding from the external os. There is marked necrosis. The patient was in her 12th week of pregnancy. (**b**) An exophytic tumor with a large deeply infiltrative component, involving most of the thickness of the cervical wall. The tumor extends to the upper part of the endocervical canal.

of lymphovascular space, confluence, multifocality, and distance from margins. In assessing the latter at the time of frozen section, either ink or cauterized epithelium should be visualized to assure the completeness of the section examined.

Key Features of Microinvasive (Superficially Invasive) Squamous Carcinoma
- Depth 3 mm or less (Invasion of 3–5 mm is classified as Stage IA2)
- Width 7 mm or less
- No capillary lymphatic space involvement (Not included in FIGO definition)
- No grossly visible lesion

Invasive Squamous Cell Carcinoma

These neoplasms can have an exophytic or endophytic pattern of growth; the latter commonly infiltrates the surrounding tissues (Figs. 4.17 and 4.18). Microscopically, most tumors are

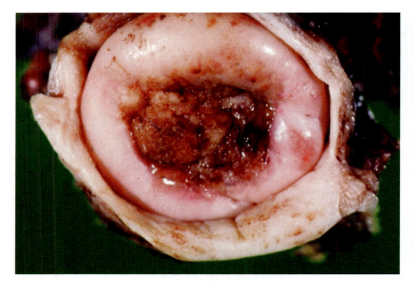

FIGURE 4.18 Invasive squamous cell carcinoma. An ulcerative lesion with irregular hemorrhagic and necrotic surface, involving most of the circumference of the cervix.

moderately differentiated large-cell nonkeratinizing type (Fig. 4.19). Keratinizing neoplasms are less common (Fig. 4.20). Small-cell type of squamous cell carcinoma is the least differentiated of the squamous cell line (Fig. 4.21). Invasive carcinomas often show variation in the pattern of growth, cell type, and degree of cellular differentiation. The infiltrating nests induce desmoplastic response in the stroma, associated with infiltration by inflammatory cells and necrosis. Determination of the tumor type may be hindered by necrosis, since the naked nuclei are difficult to differentiate from those of small cell carcinoma (Fig. 4.22). Tumor stage, which primarily relates to tumor size and extent, is considered to be the most important prognostic indicator. The presence of local or lymphatic invasion is also a significant prognostic factor. Increasing depth of invasion correlates with nodal spread and diminished progression-free interval.

Cervical carcinomas can directly invade the parametrial tissue, uterine corpus, vagina, bladder, and/or rectum. The complete

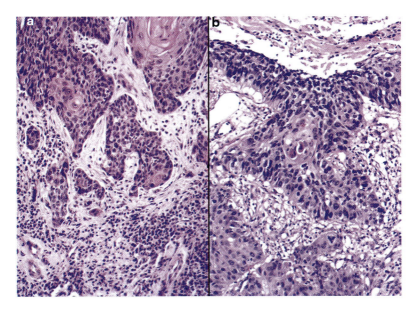

FIGURE 4.19 Invasive squamous carcinoma. (**a**) Nests of malignant squamous cells deeply invade the cervical stroma. The nests are irregular in shape and size, and they elicit a desmoplastic stromal response (H&E, medium power). (**b**) Ulceration, necrosis and inflammation are common features in invasive cancer, and are the source of the "tumor diathesis" observed in smears from such patients (H&E, medium power).

evaluation of such margins is deferred for permanent sections after formalin fixation, but frozen sections of specific areas of concern from these margins may be requested by surgeons to assure adequacy of the resection.

Lymphatic spread of cervical cancer usually occurs in an orderly stepwise fashion involving first nodes on the pelvic sidewall to the common iliac and the paraaortic lymph nodes. The obturator lymph node is the most frequently involved pelvic lymph node. Occasionally, a suspicious or a sentinel node identified by technetium 99 and dye is also submitted for intraoperative consultation. Sensitivity and specificity of the sentinel node frozen biopsy in cervical cancers are currently reported to be 95.2 and 80%, respectively. A touch preparation of lymph nodes and staining of the cytologic smear may help in confirming the presence of tumor

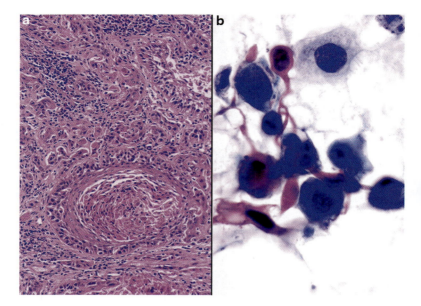

FIGURE 4.20 Keratinizing squamous cell carcinoma. (a) The invasive nests of well differentiated squamous cells show central keratinization. (b) Touch preparation of a pelvic lymph node showing high N/C ratio, hyperchromasia, and "tadpole" cytoplasmic tails (Papanicolaou stain, high power, oil).

cells (see Fig. 4.20). However, this should be used in conjunction with histologic examination which should include multiple cross sections of the sentinel node. In addition to lymphatic spread, squamous cell carcinoma may also spread by hematogenous route to the lungs, liver, and bones.

Differential Diagnostic Considerations

Establishing the presence of vascular involvement may be problematic, particularly in microinvasive lesions with only a few small nests of neoplastic cells. These nests often retract from the surrounding stroma due to fixation and freezing, and the resulting spaces are lined by flattened stromal cells. True capillary lymphatic space invasion is usually in the form of well defined nests with smooth outer margins, and their shape fits into the contour of the vascular space, with no evidence of desmoplastic reaction in the stroma immediately surrounding the vessel. Endothelial markers

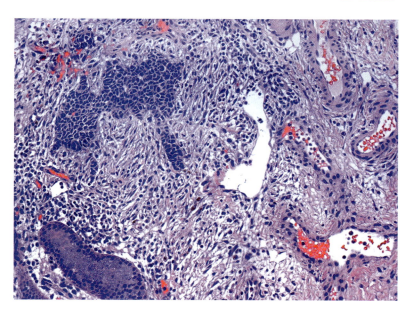

FIGURE 4.21 Small cell carcinoma. Irregularly shaped nests of poorly differentiated squamous cells, with minimal amounts of basophilic cytoplasm. Presence of foci of moderately differentiated squamous cells help in differentiating these from small cell neuroendocrine tumors, although immunostains on permanent sections may be necessary (H&E, medium power).

such as Ulex, CD 31, or D2-40 may be necessary to differentiate flattened stromal cells from true endothelial cells.

Poorly differentiated small cell variant can also present a diagnostic problem since its morphology is similar to that of small cell neuroendocrine carcinoma, particularly if there is tumor necrosis. Focal immunoreactivity to neuroendocrine markers may be seen in some cells in tumors other than neuroendocrine neoplasms. However, the differentiation between these two neoplasms is not critical at the time of surgery, since both behave aggressively, and should be deferred to routine processing and using immunostains such as CD56, synaptophysin, and chromogranin.

Verrucous carcinoma is highly differentiated and exhibits minimal cytologic atypia. It should be differentiated from condyloma acuminatum, as previously discussed under "Vulva" (see Chap. 2).

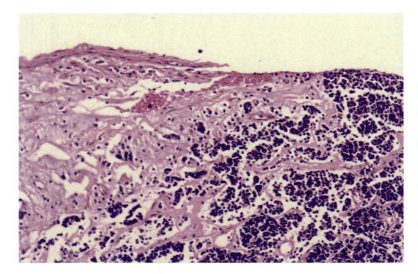

FIGURE 4.22 Extensive necrosis in an invasive carcinoma. The necrotic cells have lost the cytoplasm, leaving naked nuclei that are difficult to categorize accurately at the time of intraoperative consultation (H&E, medium power).

ADENOCARCINOMA

Adenocarcinomas represent 20–25% of cervical cancers. Human papillomavirus serotypes 16, 18, 45, 59, and 33 account for 94% of the serotypes found in these glandular malignancies. Adenocarcinomas are treated in a similar fashion as squamous cell carcinomas. If fertility is not an issue, hysterectomy is performed. If fertility is desired, cone biopsy with negative margins is considered adequate treatment for patients with AIS or invasive adenocarcinomas with a depth of invasion of 3 mm or less. The cone biopsy should be a cold knife procedure. Loop excisions obscure the depth of invasion and the assessment of margins is difficult due to cautery artifact. Patients with stage IA1 with lymphovascular invasion and stages IA2 and IB1 can be treated with radical trachelectomy and laparoscopic pelvic lymphadenectomy. Evaluation of the endocervical margin on cone biopsies or trachelectomy specimens for AIS is critical because it can alter the immediate surgical management.

Several types of adenocarcinoma are encountered in the cervix (Table 4.2). The most common are endocervical and intestinal

TABLE 4.2 Histologic types of cervical adenocarcinoma.

- Mucinous adenocarcinoma (60%)
  Endocervical type
  Intestinal (goblet cell)
- Endometrioid adenocarcinoma (30%)
- Minimal deviation adenocarcinoma (1%)
- Villoglandular adenocarcinoma (rare)
- Clear cell adenocarcinoma (2–4%)
- Serous adenocarcinoma (1%)
- Adenosquamous carcinoma (4%)

adenocarcinomas, both of which are mucinous tumors. As in squamous cell cancer, adenocarcinomas can be intraepithelial (adenocarcinoma in situ) or invasive tumors.

Glandular Intraepithelial Neoplasia

This entity is being recognized more frequently and the criteria for cytologic detection and histologic features have been better characterized recently. It includes adenocarcinoma in situ (AIS) as well as glandular dysplasia, although the concept of low- and high-grade dysplasia is not universally accepted. Most cases are only detected as a result of an abnormal smear that is followed by endocervical sampling to identify the nature and source of the abnormal glandular cells. The characteristic features of AIS include cell crowding with stratification, nuclear enlargement, nuclear hyperchromasia, mitosis, and apoptosis (Figs. 4.23 and 4.24). The role of frozen section is usually limited to ensuring a clear margin in the follow-up conization specimen if the patient desires conservative therapy. Atypical cytologic changes at the endocervical margin that are not diagnostic of AIS can be reported as glandular atypia and final diagnosis deferred for permanent sections with immunohistochemical stains, if necessary. In these cases where the status of the endocervical margin is uncertain, the surgeon may excise additional endocervical or lower uterine segment tissue. Patients with involved margins have a high incidence of residual adenocarcinoma in situ, requiring further surgery. Hysterectomy is performed in those patients for whom fertility preservation is not an issue. A repeat cone or trachelectomy is performed when there is a desire to preserve fertility.

84 FROZEN SECTION LIBRARY

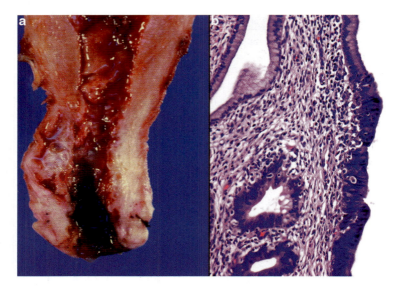

FIGURE 4.23 Glandular intraepithelial neoplasia (adenocarcinoma in situ). (**a**) Hysterectomy showing lush endocervical tissue with hemorrhage. The endocervix showed adenocarcinoma in situ, but there was no evidence of invasive adenocarcinoma (H&E, medium power). (**b**) There is nuclear hyperchromasia and crowding, associated with loss of cytoplasmic vacuolization in the two lower glands. The surface columnar cells show similar changes (H&E, medium power).

Key Histologic Features of AIS
- Cellular crowding with stratification
- Nuclear enlargement and nuclear hyperchromasia with coarse chromatin pattern
- Mitosis at the apical pole of the cell and apoptosis
- Preserved gland architecture or papillary/ cribriform intraglandular growth
- Gland–stromal interface is smooth and well demarcated

Invasive Adenocarcinomas

Invasive glandular neoplasms can be exophytic and polypoid, or endophytic and deeply infiltrative (Figs. 4.25 and 4.26). The differentiation between the various histopathologic types of adenocarcinoma is rarely an issue that needs to be settled at the time of surgery by frozen section, when adequate sampling is not feasible, and results do not have an impact on the course of surgery. A detailed discussion

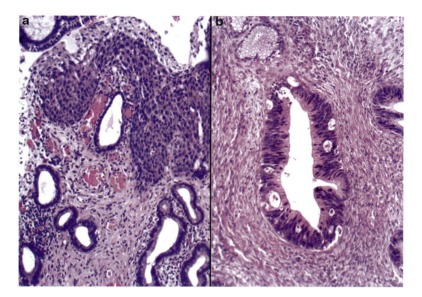

FIGURE 4.24 Glandular intraepithelial neoplasia and squamous CIN III. (a) Low power view showing squamous carcinoma in situ associated with atypical endocervical glands (H&E, low power). (b) A higher power view of a gland with nuclear enlargement, hyperchromasia and crowding, stratification and loss of cytoplasmic vacuoles (H&E, medium power).

of the various types is beyond the scope of this text, but a discussion of specific aspects as they relate to intraoperative consultation is appropriate.

Mucinous Adenocarcinoma

Mucinous adenocarcinoma is the most common type of cervical adenocarcinoma. It is divided into three subtypes: endocervical, intestinal, and signet ring. The endocervical type is the most common and the neoplastic cells resemble endocervical cells with eosinophilic or mucinous cytoplasm. Nuclear atypia, pseudostratification, loss of polarity, hyperchromasia, frequent mitosis, and apoptosis are present (Fig. 4.27). The intestinal-type adenocarcinoma is the second most common type, and is characterized by the presence of goblet cells and, less frequently, argentaffin and Paneth cells (Fig. 4.28). Signet ring type is rare and usually seen as a component of endocervical- or intestinal-type adenocarcinoma (Fig. 4.29).

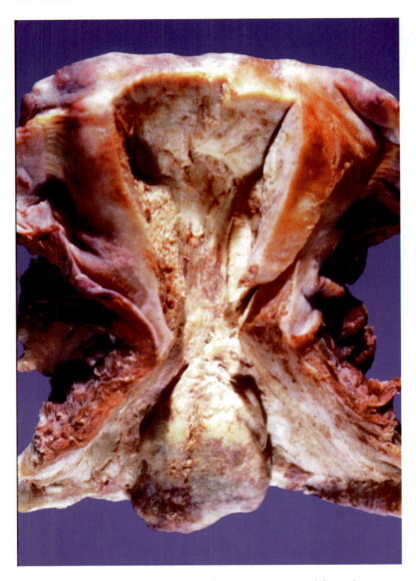

FIGURE 4.25 Adenocarcinoma. The bulky tumor originated from the upper part of the endocervical canal and filled the distended canal. See also Fig. 4.26 from the same hysterectomy specimen. From Ramzy I. Essentials of gynecologic and obstetric pathology. Norwalk: Appleton Century Crofts; 1983. p. 131. Used with permission.

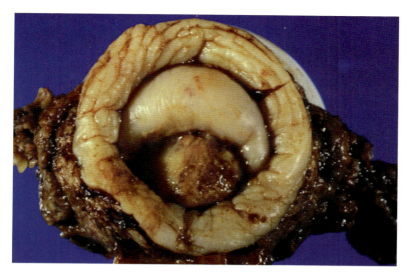

FIGURE 4.26 Adenocarcinoma. The tumor protruded from the external os and showed surface ulceration. From Ramzy I. Essentials of gynecologic and obstetric pathology. Norwalk: Appleton Century Crofts; 1983. p.131. Used with permission.

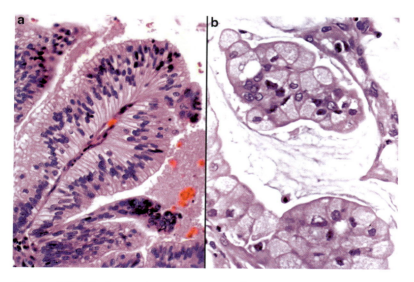

FIGURE 4.27 Mucinous adenocarcinoma, endocervical type (**a**) Tall columnar cells with clear cytoplasm and stratification and forming papillary structures. (**b**) The similarity of these cells to endocervical cells rather than goblet cells is evident. Compare with Fig. 4.28 (H&E, medium power).

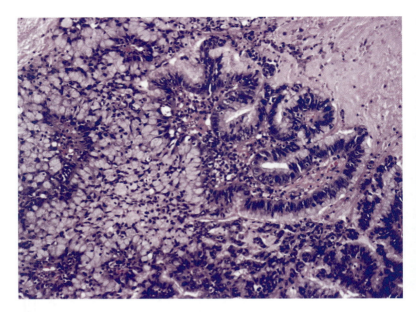

FIGURE 4.28 Mucinous adenocarcinoma, intestinal type. The neoplastic cells have a goblet-type pattern (H&E, medium power).

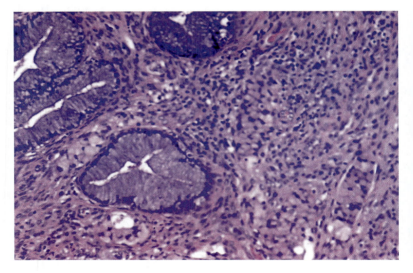

FIGURE 4.29 Mucinous adenocarcinoma, signet ring type. There is diffuse infiltration of the subepithelial stroma by nests as well as isolated signet ring cells (H&E, medium power).

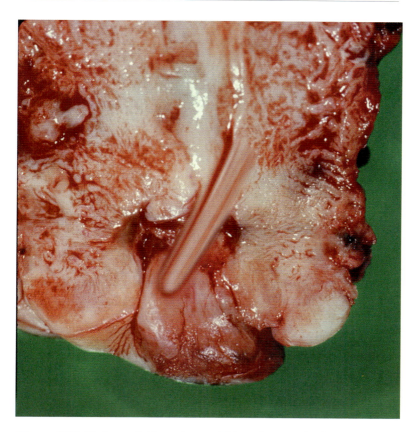

FIGURE 4.30 Endometrioid carcinoma. This endocervical adenocarcinoma was associated with endometriosis of the cervical tissues.

Key Histologic Features of Mucinous Adenocarcinoma
- Complex gland architecture with cribriform, microglandular, solid or papillary growth patterns
- Columnar cells with hyperchromatic, enlarged nuclei, and eosinophilic or mucinous cytoplasm
- Frequent mitoses and apoptotic bodies
- Infiltrative, expansile, or exophytic invasive patterns
- Desmoplastic stroma and occasional pools of mucin

Endometrioid Adenocarcinoma

The endometrioid type of cervical adenocarcinoma has a propensity to arise higher in the endocervical canal and can be difficult to determine if the site of origin is the endocervix or endometrium, in view of similar histomorphology (Figs. 4.30 and 4.31). Examination

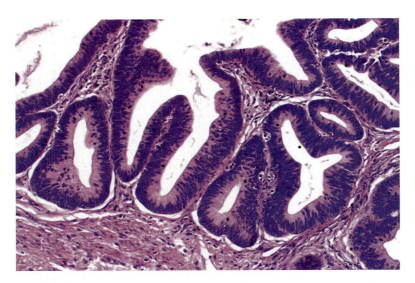

FIGURE 4.31 Endometrioid carcinoma. Note the tubulovillous architecture and lining by tall columnar cells, with elongated nuclei and moderate amounts of amphophilic cytoplasm. There is no evidence of mucinous secretion (H&E, medium power).

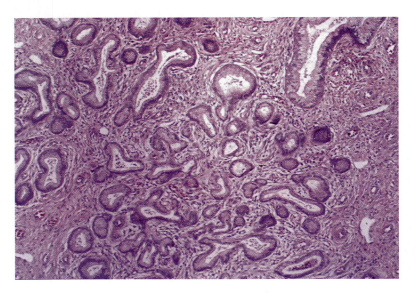

FIGURE 4.32 Minimal deviation adenocarcinoma. Although there is minimal nuclear atypia, the glands are irregular in size and shape, and they are seen within muscle deeper than the level of the normal endocervical glands/clefts. Desmoplasia, if present, can be a helpful feature (H&E, low power).

TABLE 4.3 Sources of diagnostic problems related to endocervix.

- Diathermy effects
- Tubal metaplasia
- Endometriosis
- Endometrioid metaplasia
- Microglandular hyperplasia
- Sampling of lower uterine segment
- Inflammation and repair
- Site of previous biopsy or surgery

of the junction of the endocervical canal and lower uterine segment becomes critical in this determination. However, this can be deferred to permanent section, since surgical management of lesions involving the cervix is essentially the same, regardless of the exact origin.

Minimal Deviation Adenocarcinoma

This tumor often presents a diagnostic challenge at the time of frozen section since it is highly differentiated and lacks cytologic atypia. The tumor may form a polypoid mass or ulcerate like other adenocarcinomas, or it may infiltrate a grossly unremarkable cervix. Unlike reactive glands which are near the surface, the mucinous glands of Minimal Deviation Adenocarcinoma (MDA) are deeply invasive (>8 mm deep), seen in muscle and near large blood vessels, and perivascular or perineural invasion may be encountered. These glands vary in size, have complex architectural pattern, and often run parallel to the surface (Fig. 4.32).

Differential Diagnostic Considerations

Several benign lesions of the cervix can appear highly atypical on frozen sections, and may be misinterpreted as evidence of involvement of the endocervical margin by adenocarcinoma (Table 4.3).

Cauterization of the endocervical margin, such as in the top hat component of cone biopsies, alters the columnar cells. These become elongated cells with dark nuclei similar to squamous cells and thus raise the possibility of evidence of a residual focus of AIS. This change, unlike true AIS, affects the entire surface epithelium; the spindled nuclei have poorly preserved chromatin, and the cytoplasm is cloudy (see Fig. 4.11). *Tubal metaplasia* shows nuclear crowding, but the presence of an occasional ciliated cell and lack of prominent nuclear pleomorphism help differentiate it from AIS.

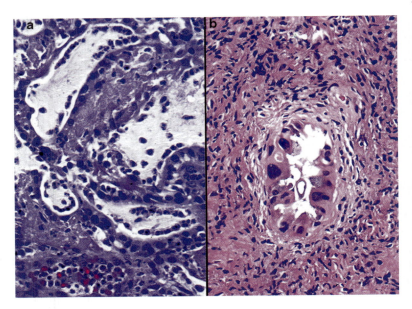

FIGURE 4.33 Reactive atypia (a) Repair associated with inflammation may result in glandular cell atypia. The nuclei may be enlarged but they usually lack hyperchromasia and cell stratification. Their chromatin is often smudged (H&E, medium power). (b) Radiotherapy may induce atypia in the glandular epithelium, with nuclear enlargement, and hyperchromasia. There is homogenization of the chromatin, vacuolization within nuclei, and a concomitant cytoplasmic enlargement (H&E, medium power).

Pleomorphic nuclei are not usually encountered in endometriosis or endometrial metaplasia unless there is hemorrhage. *Other benign processes* that may mimic AIS include endocervicitis, Arias Stella reaction, and atypia secondary to therapy effect such as radiotherapy (Fig. 4.33). Questionable cases that are not diagnostic of AIS should be reported as glandular atypia and the final diagnosis deferred until well-oriented permanent sections are examined. In such cases, the surgeon may excise additional endocervical or lower uterine segment tissue.

Progestational agents can induce microglandular hyperplasia of the endocervical glands, with nuclear hyperchromasia, some nuclear enlargement, and cytoplasmic vacuolization. Unlike adenocarcinoma, these glands are small, ill-defined, and are often associated with inflammatory cell infiltrate and squamous metaplasia (Fig. 4.34).

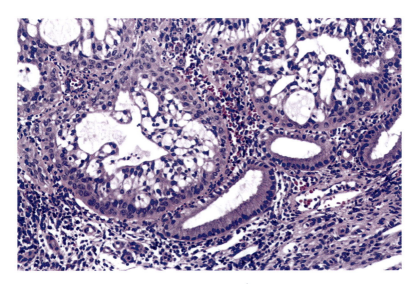

FIGURE 4.34 Microglandular hyperplasia. Note small glands, poor definition of the glands, subnuclear vacuoles, and presence of inflammatory cells. Squamous metaplasia is often closely associated with such foci (H&E, medium power).

In addition, other benign processes that may simulate cervical adenocarcinoma include tunnel clusters, mesonephric hyperplasia, and endocervical glandular hyperplasia, as well as diffuse laminar endocervical glandular hyperplasia. Most of these benign mimics display some lobular arrangement of the glands, lack significant cellular atypia, mitotic activity, or desmoplastic stromal response. On the contrary, invasive adenocarcinomas have deeply infiltrative glands, more significant nuclear atypia, and mitotic activity, as well as desmoplastic stromal response.

NEUROENDOCRINE CARCINOMAS

These uncommon neoplasms account for less than 5% of all cervical carcinomas. They include small cell carcinomas (which may also represent a poorly differentiated squamous or adenocarcinoma), carcinoid tumors, and large cell neuroendocrine tumors. Neuroendocrine carcinomas display aggressive behavior, are often ulcerated, necrotic, and more infiltrative than squamous cell carcinomas or adenocarcinomas. The diagnosis can be suggested at

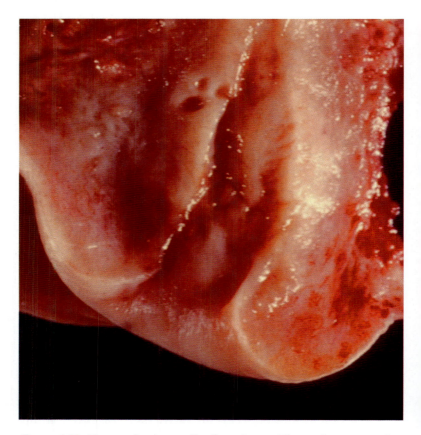

FIGURE 4.35 Neuroendocrine small cell carcinoma. The cervix appears to be indurated and thickened due to deep infiltration of the wall by the pale area of neoplastic cells. The lesion is predominantly endocervical and shows no evidence of ulceration.

the time of frozen section, based on nuclear features of "salt and pepper" chromatin, and scant cytoplasm (Figs. 4.35 and 4.36). In some instances, definitive classification and differentiation from other small cell malignancies, such as lymphomas, require immunohistochemical staining of permanent sections (Fig. 4.37). It is also important to note that focal neuroendocrine differentiation may be encountered in other tumors such as adenocarcinoma or squamous cell carcinoma.

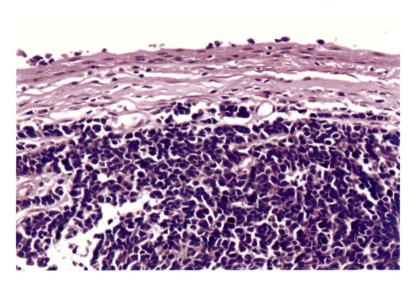

FIGURE 4.36 Neuroendocrine small cell carcinoma. Small cells with scant cytoplasm and relatively large nuclei. There are no attempts at glandular or squamous differentiation. However, neuroendocrine tumors may be associated with squamous or glandular carcinomas (H&E, medium power).

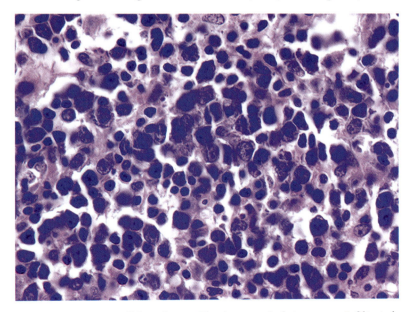

FIGURE 4.37 Large cell lymphoma: The deep cervical tissues are infiltrated by lymphocytes that proved to be monoclonal by flow cytometry. The differential diagnosis includes small cell carcinoma, severe chronic cervicitis, and follicular cervicitis (H&E, high power).

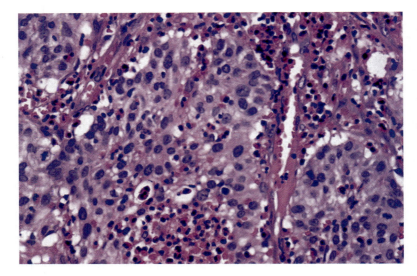

FIGURE 4.38 Glassy cell carcinoma. The neoplastic cells have abundant glassy eosinophilic cytoplasm. The dense eosinophilic stromal response helps to differentiate this tumor from squamous cell neoplasms (H&E, high power).

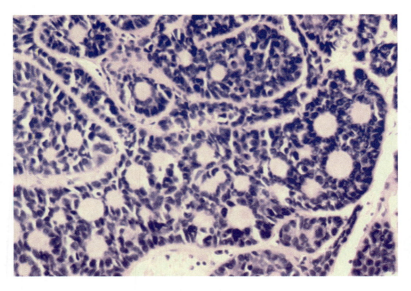

FIGURE 4.39 Adenoid cystic carcinoma: The neoplastic cells are arranged in sheets with cribriform pattern similar to adenoid cystic carcinomas of salivary glands. The spaces contain basement membrane like material (H&E, medium power).

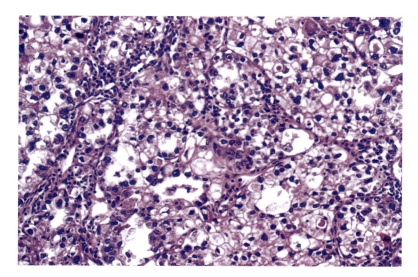

FIGURE 4.40 Clear cell carcinoma: The neoplastic cells have central or eccentric nuclei surrounded by clear cytoplasm (H&E, medium power).

UNCOMMON NEOPLASMS

Glassy cell carcinoma is a rare type of cervical malignancy consisting of large cells with eosinophilic ground-glass like cytoplasm. The presence of an eosinophilic stromal infiltrate helps differentiating it from squamous cell carcinoma. The tumor may show focal glandular or squamous differentiation (Fig. 4.38). *Adenoid cystic carcinoma* has been reported in the cervix and its histogenesis is not clear. The cells are bland, with scant cytoplasm and high N/C ratio. They are arranged in cords and nests, similar to those encountered in salivary glands (Fig. 4.39). Other carcinomas such as verrucous carcinoma and clear cell carcinoma (Fig. 4.40) are discussed in detail in Chaps. 2 and 3.

Embryonal rhabdomyosarcoma is extremely rare in the cervix. It originates in the cervical sub-epithelial müllerian stroma, usually in children or young adults, and is similar to those originating in the vagina. *Carcinosarcoma*, on the other hand, affects older patients, usually in their 60s. The tumors show a variety of homologous or heterologous elements, and require extensive sampling to reveal the different elements present (Fig. 4.41). They will be discussed further in Chap. 5, together with other stromal and smooth muscle neoplasms of the uterine body. Metastases from genital tract organs or from other primary sites occasionally involve the cervix (Fig. 4.42).

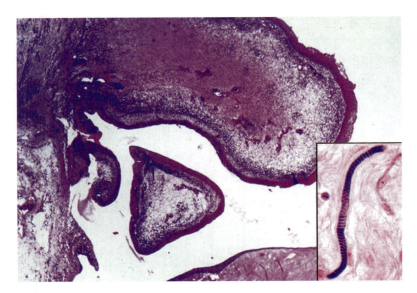

FIGURE 4.41 Rhabdomyosarcoma: This tumor was encountered in a 19 year old girl. The polypoid mass shows loose and dense mesenchymal tissues, with a dense "cambium" layer under the epithelium. Other areas of the tumor showed islands of cartilage and undifferentiated mesenchymal cells (H&E, low power). Inset shows rhabdomyoblasts with cross striations (H&E, medium power).

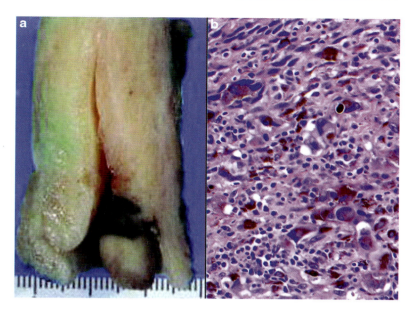

FIGURE 4.42 Malignant melanoma, metastatic: (**a**) Hysterectomy specimen showing a pigmented mass involving most of the upper cervical canal. (**b**) The neoplasm consists mostly of spindle cells with focal *brown* melanin pigmentation (H&E, medium power).

REFERENCES

Anderson WA, Leiser R, Taylor PT, Thorton Jr WN. The Frozen section analysis of conization. A reappraisal of the ends and means. Diagn Gynecol Obstet. 1982;4:251–4.

Baker P, Oliva E. A practical approach to intraoperative consultation in gynecological pathology. Int J Gynecol Pathol. 2008;27:353–65.

Benedet JL, Anderson GH. Stage IA carcinoma of the cervix revisited. Obstet Gynecol. 1996;87:1052–9.

Berek JS, Hacker NF, editors. Berek & Hacker's practical gynecologic oncology. 5th ed. Philadelphia, PA: Lippincott Williams & Wilkins; 2009.

Bosch FX, de Sanjose S. Human papillomavirus and cervical cancer-burden and assessment of causality. J Natl Cancer Inst Monogr. 2003;31:3–13.

Chenevert J, Tetu B, Plante M, et al. Indication and method of frozen section in vaginal radical trachelectomy. Int J Gynecol Pathol. 2009;28:480–8.

Clements PB, Young RH. Atlas of gynecologic surgical pathology. Philadelphia, PA: WB Saunders; 2000.

Crum CP, Nucci MR, Lee KR, editors. Diagnostic gynecologic and obstetric pathology. Philadelphia, PA: Elsevier Saunders; 2011.

DiSaia PJ, Creasman WT. Clinical gynecologic oncology. 7th ed. Philadelphia, PA: Mosby-Elsevier; 2007.

Fanfani F, Ludovisi M, Zannoni GF, et al. Frozen section examination of pelvic lymph nodes in endometrial and cervical cancer: accuracy in patients submitted to neoadjuvant treatments. Gynecol Oncol. 2004;94: 779–84.

Giuntoli RL, Winburn KA, Silverman B, et al. Frozen section evaluation of cervical cold knife cone specimens is accurate in the diagnosis of microinvasive squamous cell carcinoma. Gynecol Oncol. 2003;91:280–4.

Gu M, Lin F. Efficacy of cone biopsy of the uterine cervix during frozen section for the evaluation of cervical intraepithelial neoplasia grade 3. Am J Clin Pathol. 2004;122:383–8.

Hannigan EV, Simpson JS, Dillard EA, Dinh TV. Frozen section evaluation of cervical conization specimens. J Reprod Med. 1986;31:11–4.

Hasenburg A et al. Evaluation of lymph nodes in squamous cell carcinoma of the cervix: touch imprint cytology versus frozen section histology. Int J Gynecol Cancer. 1999;9:337–41.

Hoffman MS, Collins E, Roberts WS, et al. Cervical conization with frozen section before planned hysterectomy. Obstet Gynecol. 1993;82:394–8.

Hoskins W, Perez CA, Young RC. Principles and practice of gynecologic oncology. 3rd ed. Philadelphia, PA: Lippincott William & Wilkins; 2000.

Ismiil N, Ghorab Z, Covens A, et al. Intraoperative margin assessment of the radical trachelectomy specimen. Gynecol Oncol. 2009;113:42–6.

Kaufman RH. Frozen section evaluation of the cervical conization specimen. Clin Obstet Gynecol. 1967;10:838–52.

Lecuru F, Neji K, Robin F, et al. Microinvasive carcinoma of the cervix: rationale for conservative treatment in early squamous cell carcinoma. Eur J Gynaecol Oncol. 1997;18:465–70.

Neiger R, Bailey SA, Wall 3rd AM, et al. Evaluating cervical cone biopsy specimens with frozen sections at hysterectomy. J Reprod Med. 1991;36: 103–7.

Noriaki S, Chikara S, Naoki T, et al. Incidence and distribution pattern of pelvic and paraaortic lymph node metastasis in patients with Stage IB, IIA and IIB cervical carcinoma treated with radical hysterectomy. Cancer. 1999;85:1547–54.

Nucci MR, Oliva E. Gynecologic pathology. London: Elsevier Churchill Livingstone; 2009 (volume in the series foundations in diagnostic pathology).

Nucci MR. Symposium part III: tumor-like glandular lesions of the uterine cervix. Int J Gynecol Pathol. 2002;21:347–59.

Östör AG, Duncan A, Quinn M, Rome R. Adenocarcinoma in situ of the uterine cervix: an experience with 100 cases. Gynecol Oncol. 2000;79: 207–10.

Park K, Oslow R, Sonoda Y. Frozen section evaluation of cervical adenocarcinoma at time of radical trachelectomy: pathologic pitfalls and the application of an objective scoring system. Gynecol Oncol. 2008;110:316–23.

Rojat-Habib MC, Cravello L, Bretelle F, et al. Value of endocervical margin examination of conization specimens. Prospective study conducted on 150 patients. Gynecol Obstet Fertil. 2000;28:929–30.

Robboy SJ, Anderson MC, Russell P. Pathology of the female reproductive tract. London: Churchill Livingstone; 2002.

Sakuragi N, Satoh C, Takeda N, et al. Incidence and distribution pattern of pelvic and paraaortic lymph node metastasis in patients with Stage IB, IIA and IIB cervical carcinoma treated with radical hysterectomy. Cancer. 1999;85:1547–54.

Rock JA, Johns III HW. TeLinde's operative gynecology. 10th ed. Philadelphia, PA: Lippincott William & Wilkins; 2008.

Torres JE, Moorman J, Shiu A, Gyer D. Colposcopically directed conization for frozen section examination in the management of cervical intraepithelial neoplasia. J Reprod Med. 1983;28:123–5.

Van den Tillaart SAHM, Trimbos JBMZ, Dreef EJ, et al. Patterns of parametrial involvement in radical hysterectomy specimens of cervical cancer patients. Internat J Gynecol Pathol. 2011;30:185–92.

Woodford HD, Poston W, Elkins TE. Reliability of the frozen section in sharp knife cone biopsy of the cervix. J Reprod Med. 1986;31:951–3.

Zaino RJ, Ward S, Delgado G, et al. Histopathologic predictor of the behavior of surgically treated stage IB squamous cell carcinoma of the cervix. A gynecologic oncology group study. Cancer. 1992;69:1750–8.

Chapter 5
Uterine Body

Intraoperative consultations of material from the uterine body are mostly related to evaluation of specimens from hysterectomies, performed for a wide variety of reasons. These reasons will be considered first, followed by a discussion of the different specimens submitted from the operating room and the related clinical background. The last part of the chapter considers selected conditions and differential diagnostic issues associated with these entities.

REASONS FOR INTRAOPERATIVE CONSULTATION
Common indications include uterine prolapse, leiomyomas, endometrial hyperplasia, cervical cancers, and endometrial cancers (Table 5.1). The type and extent of specimen submitted depend on the indication for the operation, and handling each specimen should be tailored to provide answers to the specific questions related to this case. For myomectomy specimens, frozen sections are not usually requested unless the surgeon encounters unusual gross or clinical features that raise suspicion of the nature of the mass and its malignant potential. Endometrial curettage specimens are rarely submitted for frozen section evaluation. In some circumstances, the request is only for gross intraoperative consultation without frozen sections. However, that decision must be left to the pathologist who will have the ultimate responsibility of establishing the diagnosis.

UTERINE CORPUS SPECIMENS
The majority of specimens submitted for frozen section is in the form of hysterectomies with or without the uterine adnexa, and are sometimes accompanied by pelvic node dissections. They are performed for treatment of cervical or corpus neoplasms, as well as for non-neoplastic conditions such as hyperplasia. Other specimens

TABLE 5.1 Reasons for intraoperative consultations in the uterine body.

- Type and grade of endometrial adenocarcinoma
- Depth of invasion by endometrial carcinoma
- Extent of invasion and involvement of the cervix by endometrial cancer
- Status of pelvic lymph nodes
- Type of smooth muscle neoplasms
- Nature of stromal nodules
- Presence of peritoneal spread
- Differentiation between primary and metastatic neoplasms
- Exclude presence of chorionic villi prior to planning surgery

submitted from the corpus uteri include more limited resections such as myomectomies. Occasionally frozen section evaluation is requested for an endometrial curettage or an endometrial biopsy.

ENDOMETRIAL CURETTAGE AND ENDOMETRIAL BIOPSY

Clinical Background
Endometrial biopsies or the more extensive curettage specimens are rarely submitted for immediate intraoperative consultation. Submission of these specimens for frozen sections should be strongly discouraged if the immediate management is not going to be affected by the results. The surgeon's curiosity and the patient's anxiety are not valid reasons to freeze these specimens and increase the risk of misinterpretation. Occasionally, however, frozen section is requested in order to rule out malignancy prior to performing hysterectomy for benign disease such as a leiomyoma; if an endometrial malignancy is encountered, subsequent management may be modified. Curettage material is occasionally submitted also to rule out the presence of chorionic villi prior to performing other procedures.

Specimen Handling
Endometrial curettage specimens can present a technical challenge in view of their size, fragmented nature, and presence of blood. Freezing artifact and the loss of scant biopsy material while facing a block may hinder the ability to render a definitive diagnosis on permanent sections. There is also a distinct concern that not all fragments of an abundant curettage specimen are represented on the slides. The presence of blood clots may also result in artifactual cytologic changes in the frozen fragments, further interfering with interpretation.

Interpretation and Differential Diagnostic Considerations

Several differential diagnostic issues, such as differentiating complex atypical hyperplasia from a well-differentiated adenocarcinoma, will be discussed in this chapter. These limitations become more challenging on frozen section. A diagnosis of "Complex hyperplasia with atypia, a grade I adenocarcinoma cannot be ruled out" is appropriate in many situations, deferring the final definitive diagnosis until permanent sections of the entire curettage specimen are examined. Stromal reactions, such as those associated with exogenous progestational stimulation, may be florid and associated with nuclear atypia, necrosis, and hemorrhage; they can mimic a sarcoma on frozen section, particularly when such history is not available (refer to discussion under endometrial stromal sarcoma).

HYSTERECTOMY FOR BENIGN DISEASE

Hysterectomies or more limited resections, including endoscopic procedures, are frequently used in the management of benign diseases of the uterus. The lesions that are often encountered in the frozen section room include endometrial hyperplasia, leiomyomas, benign endometrial polyps, adenomyomas, and, less commonly, adenofibromas or other benign tumors (Fig. 5.1). Examination of

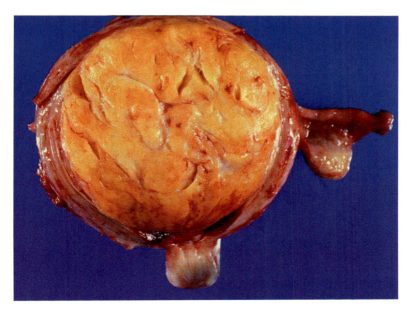

FIGURE 5.1 Hysterectomy. The uterine cavity is distended by a large lipoleiomyoma.

the uterus follows the same steps described later under hysterectomy for endometrial hyperplasia.

MYOMECTOMY

Clinical Background

Leiomyomas are the most common uterine tumors, encountered in approximately 75% of hysterectomy specimens. Myomectomies are often performed when hysterectomy is to be avoided for clinical considerations such as desire to maintain fertility or to reduce morbidity. The resected mass is usually sent for routine processing, but sometimes a frozen section evaluation is requested if the clinical manifestations are alarming, such as a rapid increase in the size.

Specimen Handling and Interpretation

On gross examination, most tumors start as intramural neoplasms; some eventually become subserous or submucosal. It is important to note if the tumor is circumscribed, as opposed to having poorly demarcated margins. If the serosa is included, the external surface should be inked. The specimen is serially sectioned to evaluate any evidence of necrosis, hemorrhage, myxoid degeneration, or areas of infarct (Fig. 5.2). Sections for frozen evaluation should include

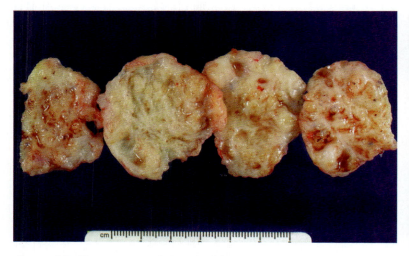

FIGURE 5.2 Myomectomy: The resected leiomyoma is serially sectioned to identify any suspicious areas of homogenization, change in color or texture that should be sampled for frozen section consultation.

any of the grossly suspicious areas that have lost the characteristic whorly pattern of a benign leiomyoma. Areas of the mass that show different color or texture should be sampled for routine processing as paraffin blocks. The criteria for interpretation of the material and the differential diagnostic issues are discussed with those of leiomyosarcoma.

ENDOMETRIAL POLYPECTOMY

Clinical Background and Specimen Handling
Most polyps are benign endometrioid type, originating from the corpus. Usually, they are not submitted for intraoperative consultations, since the evaluation does not have an impact on the planned operative procedure. Occasionally, a polypoid lesion may raise a clinical suspicion or the surgeon may want to exclude a malignancy in an unexpected lesion. The number of sections submitted for freezing depends on the size of the polyp. Large polyps are bisected and one half is frozen, leaving the other half for routine processing if possible; this ensures that part of the specimen will be adequately fixed and processed for routine examination without freezing artifact, as previously discussed under curettage specimens.

Interpretation and Differential Diagnostic Considerations
Endometrial polyps have a smooth surface but may show surface ulceration, necrosis, or hemorrhage. On cut section, cystic spaces are often visible (Fig. 5.3). Microscopically, the glands can be similar to those of proliferative, inactive, hyperplastic, or metaplastic endometrium, often with cystic dilatation. The stroma differs from the usual endometrial stroma by showing larger thick-walled blood vessels, some fibrosis, and occasionally smooth muscle (Fig. 5.4). Secretory changes may be seen in the epithelium, as well as decidual changes in the stroma, particularly if the patient received hormonal therapy for dysfunctional bleeding. Thrombosis, hemorrhage, inflammation, or ulceration may induce reactive atypia in the stromal cells that should not be interpreted as evidence of malignancy. Development of endometrioid carcinoma within an otherwise benign endometrial polyp has been reported, particularly in association with Tamoxifen treatment (Fig. 5.5). Rarely, a serous adenocarcinoma is encountered in an endometrial polyp and the malignancy may be limited to the surface of the polyp. It is important to exclude malignancies that can present as polypoid lesions, including adenocarcinoma, adenosarcoma, and other sarcomas.

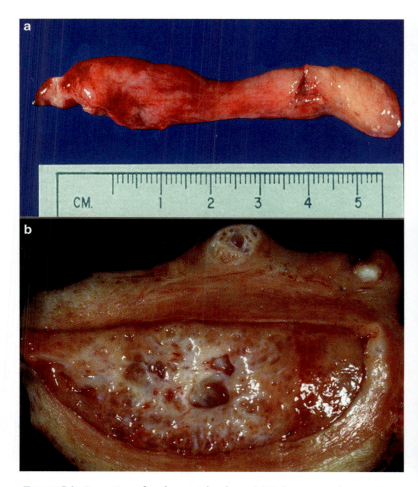

FIGURE 5.3 Resection of endometrial polyps: (a) Polypectomy for a pedunculated polyp, with necrosis at the tip. (b) Simple hysterectomy for a large sessile endometrial polyp. The 52-year-old patient presented with menorrhagia of several months duration.

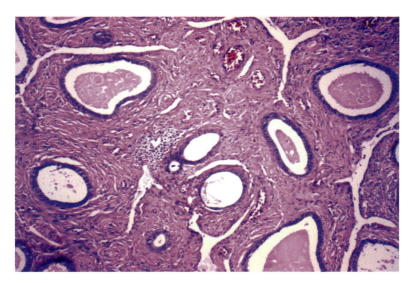

FIGURE 5.4 Endometrial polyp: The glands are often cystic and the stroma is fibrous and less cellular than the usual endometrial stroma. Thick-walled blood vessels are seen. These features help to establish the diagnosis in fragments of endometrial tissue procured by curettage (H&E, low power).

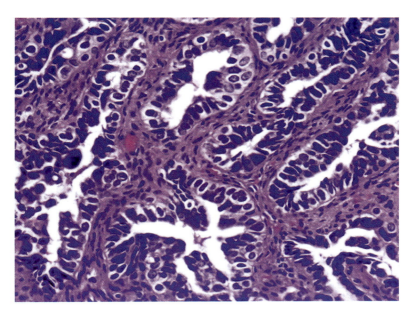

FIGURE 5.5 Endometrial polyp associated with adenocarcinoma. The patient had focal areas of endometrial glands showing nuclear pleomorphism and hyperchromasia. Malignant transformation of endometrial polyps is uncommon (H&E, high power).

HYSTERECTOMY FOR CERVICAL CANCER

Clinical Background and Types of Hysterectomy

There are several variations of abdominal hysterectomy for the management of cervical carcinoma, depending on the extent of the tumor. Although the traditional classification is into the five types listed below, the recent trend is to base the classification solely on the lateral extent of the resection, subdividing the procedures into four types, A–D.

1. *Extrafascial abdominal hysterectomy* (class I hysterectomy) consists of resection of the uterus and a small cuff of the upper vagina. It is usually performed for patients with preinvasive or microinvasive disease, if childbearing has been completed.
2. *Modified radical or extended hysterectomy* (class II hysterectomy) includes resection of the uterine body, cervix, and upper vagina, together with the medial paracervical tissues (Fig. 5.6).

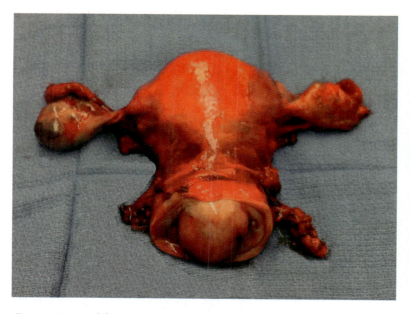

FIGURE 5.6 Modified radical hysterectomy: A hysterectomy with bilateral salpingooophorectomy. The resected specimen also includes part of the vaginal cuff and paracervical tissues. The latter should be inked at the time of receiving the specimen, particularly in areas where the tumor appear to be close to the resection margin. Slide courtesy of Dr. Yvette Williams-Brown, Houston, Texas, USA.

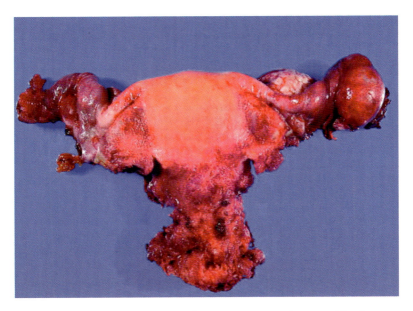

FIGURE 5.7 Radical hysterectomy for invasive cervical cancer. The laparoscopically assisted resection included the uterus, upper 25% of the vagina, uterosacral and vesicosacral ligaments, parametrium, as well as both uterine tubes and ovaries. Robotic pelvic lymphadenectomy, using the DaVinci robot, was also performed.

This procedure is performed in patients with 3–5 mm of invasion (stage IA2 cervical cancer) and for small lesions that do not distort the anatomy.
3. *Radical abdominal hysterectomy with bilateral pelvic lymphadenectomy* (class III hysterectomy) includes hysterectomy with resection of the parametrial tissues to the pelvic wall, a vaginal cuff of 2–3 cm, as well as bilateral pelvic lymphadenectomy. It is the most commonly performed operation for stage IB cervical cancer (Fig. 5.7, also Chap. 4).
4. *Extended radical hysterectomies* (class IV or V) are rarely performed because patients with large tumors that encroach on the ureter or parametrium are best treated with irradiation.
5. *Total pelvic exenteration* is performed in cases of recurrent cervical carcinomas. Such specimens include the urinary bladder, uterus with attached adnexa, vagina, and rectum. In cases where urinary bladder is included, the resection is classified as anterior

exenteration, while if rectum is included, the term posterior exenteration is used. Gross examination in these cases must include inspection of the urethral, ureteral, vaginal, and rectal margins.

Specimen Handling
The uterus is oriented using specific landmarks: the round ligaments are most anterior, and the ovaries most posterior. The peritoneum extends further inferiorly along the posterior aspect of the uterus, to cover the upper part of the vagina. Inspection of the cervix follows with description of any gross lesions. The paracervical tissue, anterior and posterior soft tissue margins as well as the vaginal cuff margin are inked. The paracervical tissue is shaved and submitted in its entirety. The margins to evaluate possibly by frozen sections include the paracervical tissues and the vaginal cuff. The uterus is bivalved, and the extent of cervical involvement, extension to vagina or lower uterine segment should be noted. If the extent of the lesion is not grossly evident, the entire cervix should be submitted for permanent sections in the same manner as a cone biopsy.

Interpretation
The interpretation of hysterectomies performed during the course of treatment of cervical cancer, the various neoplasms, and differential diagnostic issues were considered previously in Chap. 4. The evaluation of the regional lymph nodes warrants a detailed discussion below.

PELVIC LYMPH-NODE RESECTION

Clinical Background
Lymphatic drainage of the upper two-thirds of the vagina and the uterus is primarily to the obturator, internal iliac, and external iliac nodes. Evaluation of pelvic lymph nodes including right and left internal iliac, obturator, common iliac, and paraaortic nodes is performed for staging of cervical carcinomas. Metastatic carcinoma is encountered in approximately 9% of women clinically staged as early invasive cervical cancer and most frequently involve the obturator lymph nodes. Frozen section diagnosis of pelvic node metastasis has a reported sensitivity of 68% and specificity of 100%. If metastatic disease is detected by frozen section, resection of the uterus may not be performed, and alternate therapeutic modalities are used.

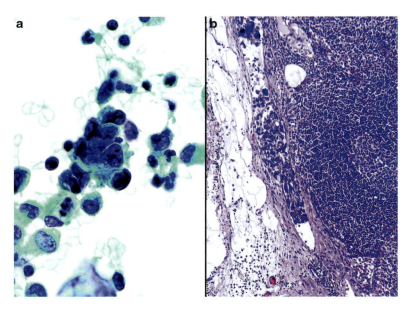

FIGURE 5.8 Metastatic carcinoma in pelvic nodes: (**a**) A pelvic lymph node imprint showing malignant cells with large pleomorphic and hyperchromatic nuclei. These cells originated from a serous papillary endometrial carcinoma (H&E, high power, oil). (**b**) Endometrioid adenocarcinoma cells in subcapsular sinuses of a pelvic node.

Specimen Handling

Cytologic imprints of the cut surface of the lymph nodes provide a sensitive, specific, and time-efficient method to diagnose nodal metastases (Fig. 5.8). In the case of squamous cell carcinoma, the technique has been reported to have a sensitivity and specificity of 90 and 100%, respectively (Hasenburg 1999). Diagnostic difficulties arise in cases where only a few atypical or suspicious cells are encountered. Occasionally, frozen sections can miss a microscopic subcapsular deposit. In order to minimize that risk, it is advisable to cut the lymph node at two different levels, both of which can be placed on the same glass slide. If more than one node is placed in the same block, they should be carefully placed on the same plane and cut to expose all nodes adequately.

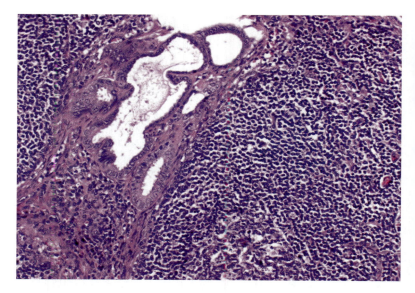

FIGURE 5.9 Benign Müllerian nest in pelvic node: The nests are often encountered in pelvic nodes in women. The well-formed glands, bland uniform nuclei, and absence of lesions within the deeper parts of the node differentiate these nests from true metastases (H&E, low power).

Interpretation and Differential Diagnostic Considerations

Benign processes including sinus histiocytosis, squamous or transitional metaplasia of the peritoneum, intranodal ectopic decidua, or hyperplasia of mesothelial inclusions within the lymph node can produce some confusion with metastatic squamous cell carcinoma. Ectopic decidua is characterized by uniform nodules of loosely cohesive cells with round vesicular nuclei and abundant cytoplasm. Metastatic squamous cell carcinoma is usually arranged as small nests of cells with eosinophilic cytoplasm and small darkly stained pleomorphic nuclei with coarse chromatin.

Similarly, benign glandular inclusions of Müllerian type, endosalpingiosis, endometriosis, and mesothelial inclusions can be encountered when sampling pelvic lymph nodes, and should be differentiated from metastatic adenocarcinoma (Fig. 5.9). The distinction is usually not difficult because of the malignant cytologic features in adenocarcinomas. The reported false negative rate of intraoperative consultation of pelvic lymph nodes ranges from 8 to 32%. Factors associated with false negative interpretation include small size of metastasis and cytomorphologic changes due to neoadjuvant therapy. False positive diagnoses are most likely due to frozen artifact and atypical endothelial cells with therapy effect.

HYSTERECTOMY FOR ENDOMETRIAL HYPERPLASIA

Clinical Background
Hysterectomy is often performed to manage some cases of endometrial hyperplasia. Specimens from patients with a preoperative diagnosis of complex atypical hyperplasia are sometimes submitted for intraoperative assessment to exclude a high-grade neoplasm. The risk of concomitant endometrial carcinoma in such patients has been reported to be 20–52%. However, most of the observed endometrial carcinomas are low stage. Only 5% of these patients have an endometrial carcinoma with more than 50% myometrial invasion. The risk of progression to carcinoma for hyperplasia without atypia is very low (2%), while a significant number of cases with atypia (23%) progress to carcinoma (Kurman).

Specimen Handling
The specimen is bivalved as previously described. The endometrial lining is carefully inspected for possible lesions or gross evidence of invasion. Frozen sections can be selected from areas of thickened endometrium or areas that are suspicious for myometrial involvement.

Interpretation
The WHO/ISGP classify hyperplasia, based on the degree of glandular architectural complexity and cytologic atypia, into: (A) simple hyperplasia and (B) complex hyperplasia; each of these can be without or with cytologic atypia. Simple hyperplasia refers to mild to moderate architectural complexity, while complex hyperplasia indicates a marked architectural complexity (Figs. 5.10 and 5.11). The second parameter, cytologic atypia, is manifested by cell crowding, enlarged rounded nuclei with prominent nucleoli, and associated with cytoplasmic eosinophilia. Pseudo or true stratification, papillary folding of the epithelium, and metaplastic changes as well as foci of adenocarcinoma may be encountered (Figs. 5.12 and 5.13). Hyperplasia may also be associated with secretory changes due to endogenous or exogenous hormonal stimulation and, occasionally, the glands may show focal ciliary metaplasia (Fig. 5.14).

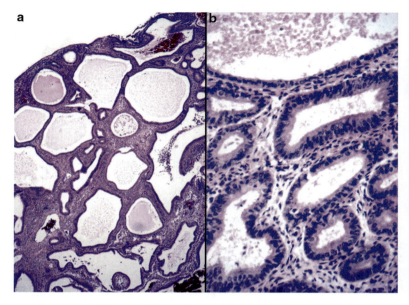

FIGURE 5.10 Endometrial hyperplasia: (a) Simple hyperplasia with large cystic glands lined by single layer of endometrial cells (H&E, low power). (b) Endometrium showing subtle changes indicative of slight complex hyperplasia without atypia, with crowded irregularly shaped glands that are lined by pseudostratified but uniform endometrial cells. The nuclei are elongated and hyperchromatic, with small or inconspicuous nucleoli (H&E, medium power).

Differential Diagnostic Considerations

Intraoperative assessment by frozen sections can identify poor prognostic pathologic factors that would necessitate surgical staging such as presence of high-grade adenocarcinomas, deep myometrial invasion, or cervical involvement. However, frozen sections can be unreliable in differentiating complex atypical hyperplasia from a noninvasive or superficially invasive well-differentiated adenocarcinoma. Features that support a diagnosis of adenocarcinoma include presence of branching papillae with cores, prominent cribriform glands, cross luminal bridges, and high-grade nuclear atypia with prominent nucleoli. Such distinction is not critical at the time of intraoperative consult, since these conditions require the same surgical management, and final definitive assessment should be deferred until extensive sampling of the endometrium is performed after proper routine fixation.

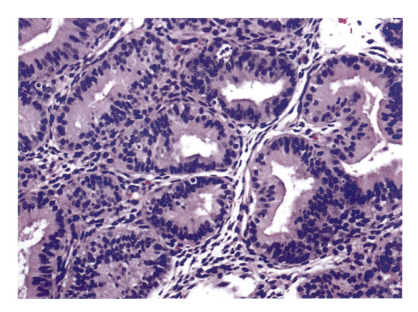

FIGURE 5.11 Endometrial hyperplasia, complex with slight atypia: Marked crowding of the glands associated with irregular shapes and enfolding. The endometrial cells show pseudostratification and some atypia. No evidence of stromal reaction in the form of histiocytes or fibrosis is seen (H&E, medium power).

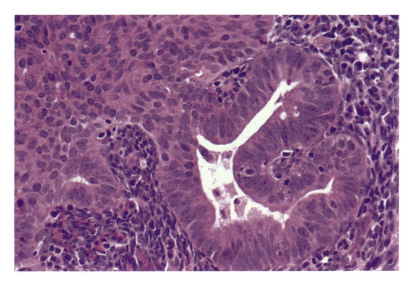

FIGURE 5.12 Endometrial hyperplasia, with atypia: The gland shows stratification, the nuclei are more *round* than those illustrated in Figs. 5.10b and 5.11 (H&E, medium power).

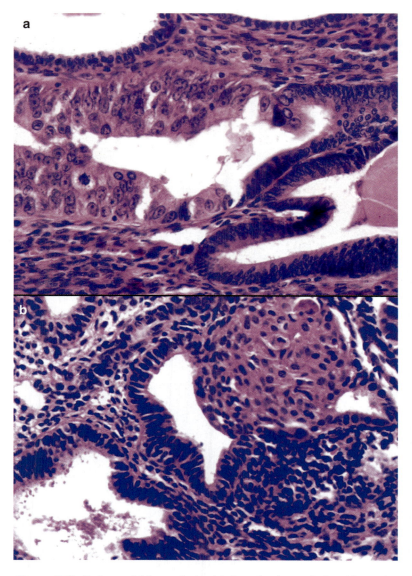

FIGURE 5.13 Endometrial hyperplasia: (**a**) Complex hyperplasia with atypia (adenocarcinoma in situ). The hyperplastic gland shows focal true stratification of the epithelium and cytoplasmic eosinophilia. The nuclei are enlarged and tend to be round. The chromatin is pale and nucleoli are prominent (H&E, high power). (**b**) Hyperplasia with morule formation. This metaplastic change should not be interpreted as evidence of malignancy. The cells of the morule have uniform nuclei that lack the features described under Fig. 5.13a (H&E, high power). From Ramzy I. Essentials in gynecologic and obstetric pathology. Norwalk: Appleton Century Crofts; 1983. p. 157. Used with permission.

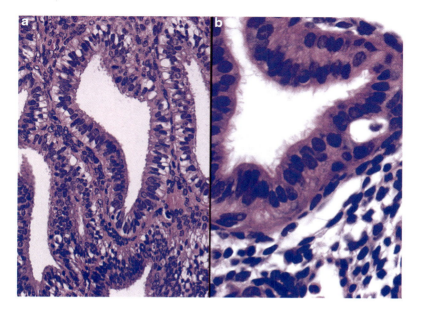

FIGURE 5.14 Endometrial hyperplasia: (**a**) Secretory changes are often the result of hormonal therapy for dysfunctional bleeding. The hyperplastic background is reflected by crowding and altered pattern of the glands differentiated this from secretory phase endometrium (H&E, medium power). (**b**) Focal ciliary metaplasia encountered in a hyperplastic endometrium without atypia (H&E, high power).

HYSTERECTOMY FOR ENDOMETRIAL CARCINOMA

Clinical Background

Hysterectomies performed for clinical stage I and II endometrial adenocarcinomas are often submitted for intraoperative consultation to determine the depth of myometrial invasion, to confirm the tumor grade, and to determine presence of endocervical involvement. The diagnosis of adenocarcinoma has been usually established by a previous curettage. The sensitivity of frozen section diagnosis in assessing deep myometrial invasion has been reported to vary from 82.7 to 85% and its specificity from 89.1 to 100% (Fishman 2000, Shim 1992). Other poor prognostic pathologic features that can be accurately determined with frozen section include histologic type cervical invasion, presence of poorly differentiated component, and adnexal involvement. Accurate assessment of these parameters allows the surgeon to correctly determine the need for pelvic and

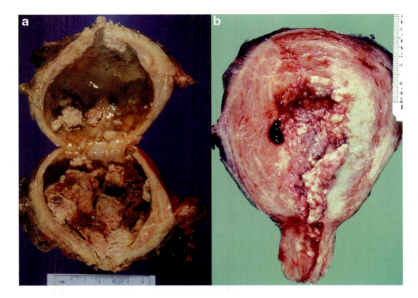

FIGURE 5.15 Endometrial adenocarcinoma: (**a**) The endometrial cavity is distended by a necrotic fungating tumor that replaced most of the endometrial lining. (**b**) Endometrial adenocarcinoma involving the entire endometrial lining and extending into the cervix.

paraaortic lymph node sampling, a procedure that adds to the duration and hence morbidity of the operation.

Pelvic node dissection may be omitted if frozen sections show that the lesion is confined to the endometrium, or a grade I endometrial carcinoma that invades less than 50% of the myometrium with no cervical extension. In all other cases, surgical staging to include lymph node sampling is performed if underdiagnosis of extrauterine disease and undertreatment is to be avoided.

Specimen Handling

After orientation of the specimen, the soft tissue resection margins around the cervix and the parametrial tissues are inked. The serosal surface is inspected for evidence of tumor extension. If present, the adnexa are removed and inspected for gross abnormalities. The uterus is bivalved into anterior and posterior halves using a probe as a guide through the endocervical canal. On gross examination, endometrial carcinomas can appear as sessile or polypoid masses and can be focal or diffuse (Figs. 5.15 and 5.16). The size, location, appearance of the tumor, and cervical extension should be recorded.

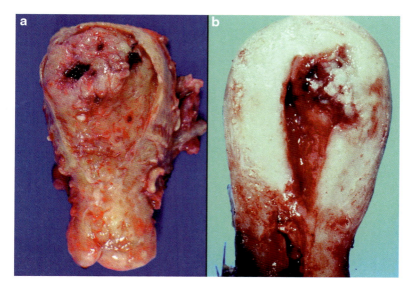

FIGURE 5.16 Endometrial adenocarcinoma: (**a**) and (**b**) Deep infiltration of the uterine wall by high-grade endometrial carcinomas, with hemorrhage and tumor necrosis. From Ramzy I. Essentials of gynecologic and obstetric pathology. Norwalk: Appleton Century Crofts; 1983. p. 182. Used with permission.

Serial transverse sections of the uterine corpus and lower uterine segment are performed. The greatest depth of tumor invasion into the myometrium must be measured. In addition, the total myometrial thickness and the distance from the tumor to the serosal surface must also be recorded. The serosa can be inked at the area of deepest myometrial invasion. The accuracy of determining depth of myometrial invasion on gross examination alone is 71%. However, gross assessment of depth of invasion becomes less accurate as the grade of the tumor increases. Depth of invasion is accurately determined on gross examination in up to 87% of grade I lesions, in 65% of grade II lesions, and in only 31% of grade III lesions. Therefore, microscopic examination is recommended to more accurately determine the depth (Fig. 5.17). In determining the maximum depth of invasion, it is important to disregard carcinomatous involvement of foci of adenomyosis. Determination of type, grade of tumor, and depth of invasion can usually be achieved with one or two full-thickness sections that include deepest point of myometrial invasion.

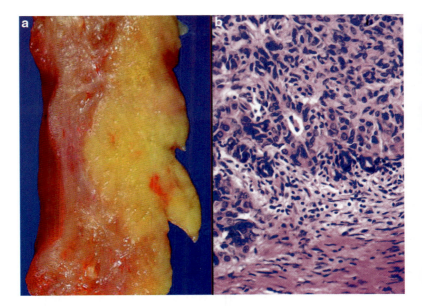

FIGURE 5.17 Endometrial adenocarcinoma: (a) The uterine tumor is sectioned at different areas to allow assessment of the depth of invasion by this yellowish-white high-grade tumor. The outer surface of the uterine wall has been inked (in *red*) at the site suspected of the deepest invasion. The depth of invasion and the thickness of the entire uterine wall at this point are reported to the surgeon (H&E, medium power). (b) A section from the outer third confirms the deep invasion of the uterine wall by solid sheets of high-grade tumor with minimal attempts at gland formation (H&E, medium power).

Cervical involvement must also be ruled out at the time of intraoperative consultation because there is a greater propensity for lymph node metastases in cases where the endocervix is involved by the tumor. If the tumor grossly approaches the lower uterine segment/endocervix it is advisable to submit sections of cervix to rule out microscopic extension.

Interpretation and Differential Diagnostic Considerations

In most instances, identification of the type of endometrial adenocarcinoma as well as degree of histology differentiation by frozen section is not difficult. Most cases submitted for intraoperative consultation have a previous curettage or biopsy-proven diagnosis of adenocarcinoma with accurate determination of type and grade of the neoplasm. However, in biopsy-proven grade I, stage I tumors the grade is increased on frozen sections in approximately 15.5% of cases. This determination will influence subsequent course of action by the surgeon. Although most types are low-grade tumors, some are considered high grade regardless of their nuclear grade or depth of myometrial invasion. These include serous papillary, undifferentiated, and clear cell carcinomas. At the time of surgical staging, 62% of patients with these unfavorable histologic subtypes have extrauterine spread of disease. Detection of an unfavorable histologic subtype at the time of frozen section, regardless of its amount, should be reported to the surgeon because its presence may alter the immediate surgical management.

A discussion of the major types and the differential diagnostic issues associated with each type is appropriate at this point. The tumors are selected on the basis of our experience in OR consults and a review of the literature. For a comprehensive discussion of all tumors, the reader is referred to the gynecologic pathology text books suggested in the references list.

Endometrioid Adenocarcinoma

Adenocarcinoma is the most common malignant neoplasm of the uterine corpus, with estimated 42,000 new cases and approximately 8,000 deaths every year in the United States; the endometrioid cell type accounts for 80% of these cases (Table 5.2). The degree of histologic differentiation is accepted as one of the most sensitive indicators of prognosis. The tumors are graded on the basis of

TABLE 5.2 Classification of endometrial carcinoma (ISGP/WHO, modified).

Endometrioid adenocarcinoma (80%)
  Typical
  Villoglandular
  With squamous differentiation
  Secretory
  Others (ciliated, oxyphilic, Sertoliform)
Serous papillary adenocarcinoma (5–10%)
Clear cell adenocarcinoma (5%)
Mucinous adenocarcinoma (<10%)
Squamous cell carcinoma (<0.5%)
Undifferentiated carcinoma
Others (hepatoid, lymphoepithelioma-like, transitional cell)

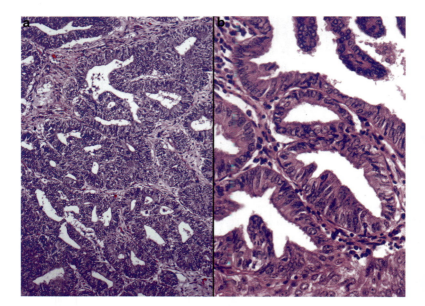

FIGURE 5.18 Endometrial adenocarcinoma, low grade: (**a**) The irregularly shaped glands are crowded, often back to back, and the epithelium is stratified. The nuclei are enlarged, more rounded, and have prominent nuclei on examination under higher magnification (H&E, low power). (**b**) Well-formed glandular structures with papillary enfolding of the neoplastic epithelium. The papillae are covered by tall columnar cells, unlike the cuboidal cells of serous papillary carcinomas (H&E, medium power). From Ramzy I. Essentials of gynecologic and obstetric pathology. Norwalk: Appleton Century Crofts; 1983. p. 185. Used with permission.

two parameters: growth pattern and nuclear morphology. Grade I tumors have less than 5% solid pattern, grade II tumors have 5–50% solid growth, and in Grade III more than 50% of the growth is solid (Figs. 5.18 and 5.19). The degree of nuclear atypia (marked pleomorphism, coarse chromatin, and prominent nucleoli) is also taken into consideration; presence of more than 25% of high-grade nuclei increases the pattern grade by one. Tumors are graded solely on the basis of their glandular component, and foci of squamous differentiation that are encountered in about 25% of adenocarcinomas are not considered as solid component. Squamous differentiation does not alter the grade of the tumor or clinical behavior (Fig. 5.20). Low grade and intermediate grade often arise in a background

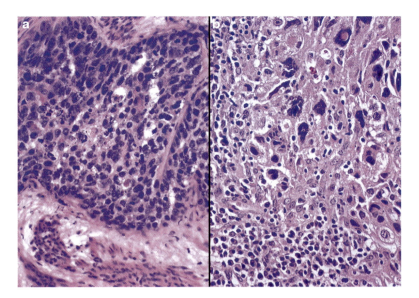

FIGURE 5.19 Endometrial adenocarcinoma, high grade: (**a**) The neoplastic cells lining the few glands have high-grade nuclei similar to those arranged in solid sheets (H&E, medium power). (**b**) This poorly differentiated carcinoma shows marked nuclear pleomorphism, necrosis, and no attempt at gland formation. The origin of the tumor from the endometrial lining of the uterus, rather than from the myometrium, may point to a carcinoma rather than a sarcoma. Immunostains are often necessary to establish the definitive classification (H&E, medium power).

of endometrial hyperplasia, thus the need for thorough sampling for routine processing. Involvement of foci of adenomyosis does not alter the prognosis or management, and is not considered as evidence of myometrial invasion.

Variants of Endometrioid Adenocarcinoma

Although mucin production is not a prominent feature of endometrioid carcinoma, occasionally it is encountered at the luminal side of neoplastic cells. Tumors with abundant mucus or glycogen are classified as "mucin-rich" or "glycogen-rich" neoplasms respectively. Villoglandular adenocarcinomas are usually low-grade neoplasms that may be pure or mixed with classic endometrioid adenocarcinoma, sharing the same behavior. They form long papillae that are lined by tall columnar cells, unlike the more cuboidal cells of

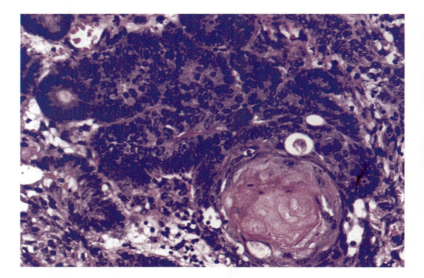

FIGURE 5.20 Endometrial adenocarcinoma, with squamous differentiation: Focal squamous differentiation with keratinization has no impact on the behavior of well-differentiated grade I adenocarcinomas. Solid sheets of epithelium indicate squamous differentiation and should not be interpreted at the time of frozen section as evidence of high-grade carcinoma. The solid sheets are intimately associated with well-formed low-grade glands and show uniform bland nuclei, unlike high-grade tumors depicted in Fig. 5.19 (H&E, medium power).

serous papillary carcinoma, a high-grade neoplasm. Endometrioid adenocarcinomas may show marked secretory pattern, cilia, a focal Sertoli-like pattern, or giant cells, all of which have no impact on the behavior; a trophoblast component, however, bespeaks of an aggressive behavior (Figs. 5.21 and 5.22).

Differentiating endometrial adenocarcinoma from adenocarcinoma of the cervix is based on gross examination of the uterus and type of normal tissues at the edge of the tumor. Features that favor endometrial origin include presence of a dominant mass in the uterine body, background hyperplastic changes of non-neoplastic endometrium, and immunoreactivity to vimentin, ER, PR, and focally with P16. In endocervical adenocarcinoma the dominant mass is in the cervix, there may be adjacent areas of cervical AIS or squamous intraepithelial lesions. Endocervical lesions are typically immunoreactive for monoclonal CEA and have diffuse P16 staining. Other differential diagnostic problems relate to serous and clear cell tumors and are discussed below.

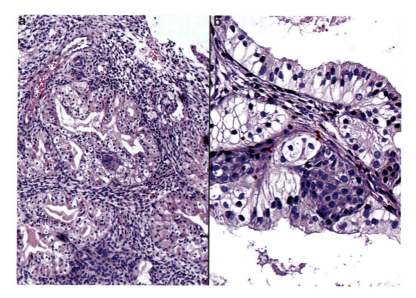

FIGURE 5.21 Endometrial adenocarcinoma, secretory: (**a**) Neoplastic cells show secretory changes in the cytoplasm. Unlike hyperplasia, the cells form glands that are back to back and have epithelial bridges across the lumen (gland within gland), in addition to solid sheets and cords (H&E, low power). (**b**) The cells are stratified with well-defined borders and clear cytoplasm. The low-grade nuclei are centrally located and lack the hobnail pattern of high-grade clear cell carcinomas (H&E, medium power).

Squamous differentiation in endometrioid carcinoma should not be misinterpreted as squamous cell carcinoma, since they have bland low-grade nuclei and are closely associated with well-differentiated neoplastic glands. Primary squamous cell carcinoma of the endometrium is rare, representing 0.5% of endometrial cancer. It shows keratinization, has high-grade nuclei, and lacks a glandular component. It should not be diagnosed in the presence of endometrial adenocarcinoma or if there is contiguity with neoplastic or normal cervical squamous epithelium.

Serous Papillary Carcinoma

This is a less common type and is considered a high-grade neoplasm regardless of its nuclear features. Its complex papillae have thick vascular cores covered by several layers of cuboidal cells. The nuclear features are almost consistently of grade III (Figs. 5.23 and 5.24a). Solid areas and deep myometrial infiltration are common features,

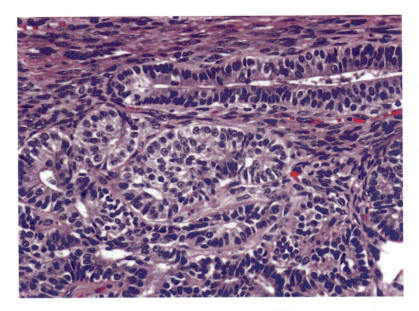

FIGURE 5.22 Endometrial adenocarcinoma, Sertoli-like pattern: Neoplastic epithelial cells arranged in cords, trabeculae, and acinar formations reminiscent of sex cords encountered in Sertoli cell tumors (H&E, medium power).

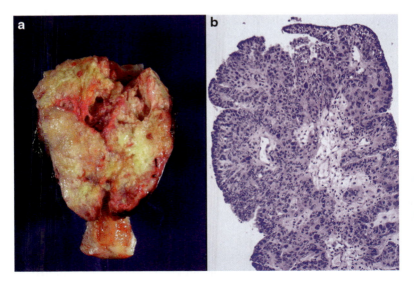

FIGURE 5.23 Endometrial adenocarcinoma, serous papillary: (a) A high-grade tumor has deeply infiltrated the uterine wall. (b) The papillae are covered by one or few layers of cuboidal cells. The high-grade nuclear features may not be discernable on frozen sections (H&E, low power).

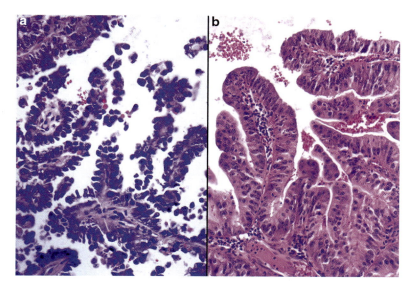

FIGURE 5.24 Papillary serous and papillary endometrioid carcinomas: (a) Permanent section of a papillary serous carcinoma, showing papillae covered by cuboidal cells with relatively scant cytoplasm. The hyperchromatic and pleomorphic nuclei characterize this high-grade neoplasm (H&E, medium power). (b) Papillary endometrioid cell adenocarcinoma cells, in contrast to those of serous carcinoma, have more abundant cytoplasm and low-grade nuclei that are less hyperchromatic and more uniform (H&E, medium power).

although occasionally a tumor may be limited to the endometrium or to an endometrial polyp. The residual endometrial lining of the uterus is usually atrophic, since the tumor occurs in an older age group than the endometrioid type. Serous papillary carcinoma has a poor prognosis even in the absence of deep myometrial invasion or lymph node metastases. Up to 75% of patients are stage III or IV at time of surgery, with evidence of nodal, ovarian, and peritoneal spread. It is often admixed with endometrioid carcinomas, but a serous component of 25% or more will portend a poor prognosis.

Serous papillary carcinoma should be differentiated from villoglandular endometrioid carcinoma. The complexity of the papillae, the tendency to tufting, the cuboidal nature of cells, and the high nuclear grade of serous carcinoma contrasts with the tall columnar cells with low-grade nuclei of villoglandular carcinoma (Fig. 5.24b). Psammoma bodies are more likely to be encountered in serous than villoglandular tumors. Furthermore, serous carcinomas are often associated with atrophic, rather than hyperplastic endometrium.

Key Histologic Features of Serous Carcinoma
- Complex papillary pattern
- Irregular thick papillae, glands, or solid architecture
- Prominent cellular budding or tufting
- Neoplastic cells exhibit marked pleomorphism, hyperchromasia, and prominent nucleoli

Key Histologic Features of Villoglandular Adenocarcinoma
- Long slender papillae with delicate fibrovascular cores
- Pseudostratified columnar cells oriented perpendicular to basement membrane
- Neoplastic cells with low-grade nuclear features
- Often admixed with areas of more conventional endometrioid adenocarcinoma

Clear Cell Carcinoma

Clear cell carcinoma is also an uncommon high-grade neoplasm that carries a similar poor prognosis to the other high-grade endometrial cancers. The tumor invades the myometrium in over 75% of cases, and it can be a component of the classic endometrioid adenocarcinoma. The neoplastic cells form papillae, tubules, and solid nests. They are polygonal with clear glycogen-rich or eosinophilic cytoplasm. Some tubulopapillary structures are lined by a single layer of cuboidal cells that protrude singly into the lumen resulting in hobnail appearance (Fig. 5.25). The nuclei are usually large, intermediate, or high grade, with prominent nucleoli. Two types of eosinophilic material are often encountered: intracytoplasmic targetoid mucin in vacuoles (signet-ring) and basement membrane deposits in the stroma of the papillae.

At time of frozen section, clear-cell carcinoma should be differentiated from lower-grade carcinomas such as secretory carcinoma and non-neoplastic conditions like Arias-Stella reaction. Secretory carcinomas consistently have low-grade nuclei and often show subnuclear vacuoles. Arias-Stella changes can be encountered in elderly patients receiving progestational therapy for endometrial adenocarcinoma. The cells show poorly preserved chromatin and decidual stromal response; a helpful clinical history may also be elicited. Differentiation from serous carcinoma is not as critical at the time of intraoperative consultation because surgical management is identical for these tumors with unfavorable histology. Serous papillary carcinoma lacks the hobnail cell pattern, hyaline deposits, and the tubulocystic spaces of clear cell carcinoma.

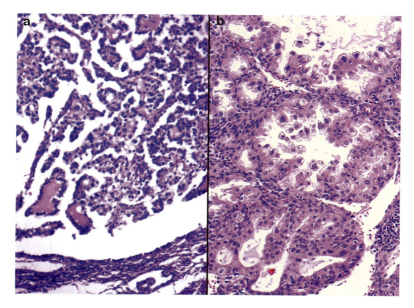

FIGURE 5.25 Endometrial adenocarcinoma, clear cell type: (**a**) The neoplastic cells are arranged as slender papillae, sheets, and clefts. They have scant, often clear cytoplasm and their high-grade nuclei often protrude into the lumen or clefts in a hobnail fashion. See also Fig. 5.13 (H&E, medium power). (**b**) Arias Stella reaction is also characterized by cells with clear cytoplasm and large nuclei that may protrude into the gland lumen. However, the degenerative bland chromatin, lack of stratification, and presence of focal decidual changes in the stroma help differentiate this from clear-cell carcinoma (H&E, medium power).

Key Histologic Features of Clear Cell Carcinoma
- Papillary, tubulocystic, and solid architecture
- Small and rounded papillae with hyalinized fibrovascular cores
- Neoplastic cells have prominent clear or eosinophilic cytoplasm
- Intracytoplasmic targetoid mucin vacuoles
- Hobnail, flat, or cuboidal tumor cells with large pleomorphic nuclei and prominent nucleoli

Key Histologic Features of Secretory Carcinoma
- Neoplastic cells with large cytoplasmic (often subnuclear) glycogen vacuoles
- Low-grade nuclear features

HYSTERECTOMY FOR SARCOMAS

Clinical Background
Treatment for uterine sarcomas often entails hysterectomy, with or without chemotherapy or radiotherapy. Uterine sarcomas are responsible for 8% of malignant neoplasms of the uterine corpus. Table 5.3 lists a modified WHO/ISGP classification of these neoplasms, although there is evidence that some sarcomas may be reclassified on the basis of recent molecular studies. Mixed epithelial / mesenchymal tumors, such as carcinosarcoma, have clinical, biologic and molecular features that are closely related to undifferentiated or high grade endometrial carcinomas, with transdifferentiation of epithelial cells to malignant mesenchymal cells (Lopez-Garcia, Palacios 2010).

Specimen Handling
Examination of hysterectomy specimens resected for sarcomas follows the same guidelines of resections for carcinomas. These tumors have a higher tendency to spread by hematogenous route, and examination of ovarian and other resected vascular structures at the time of consultation is important. Mesenchymal tumors can be bulky, requiring selective sampling. In large neoplasms, areas of necrosis, hemorrhage, variation in color or texture should be chosen for histologic examination, since this increases the

TABLE 5.3 Classification of uterine mesenchymal tumors (WHO/ISGP modified).

Endometrial stromal neoplasms
  Endometrial stromal nodule
  Endometrial stromal sarcoma, low grade
  Undifferentiated endometrial sarcoma (high grade)

Smooth muscle neoplasms
  Leiomyosarcoma, NOS and variants: epithelioid, myxoid
  Smooth muscle tumor, uncertain malignant potential
  Leiomyoma and variants (cellular, epithelioid, myxoid, atypical)

Mixed mesenchymal tumors (endometrial stromal and smooth muscle tumor)

Mixed epithelial and mesenchymal tumors
  Malignant mixed mullürian tumor (carcinosarcoma)
  Adenosarcoma
  Carcinofibroma
  Adenofibroma
  Adenomyoma and atypical polypoid variant

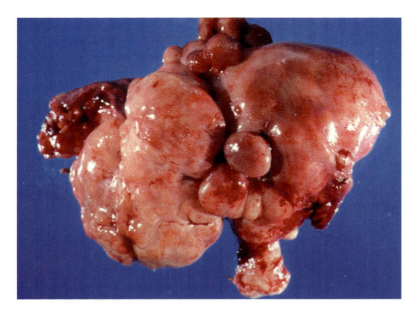

FIGURE 5.26 Smooth muscle tumor: Uterine smooth muscle neoplasms are often multiple, and cannot be all sampled for intraoperative consultation and frozen sections. Pathologists have to choose the suspicious ones for sampling, based on their gross appearance. In this case, most of the nodules proved to be benign leiomyomas, but the large mass protruding from the surface had gross features suspicious of leiomyosarcoma. They included an irregular outline, an ill-defined margin infiltrating the remainder of the myometrium. The cut surface is shown in the next Fig. 5.27a.

chance of detecting a focus of malignancy at the time of frozen. Leiomyosarcoma, when associated with multiple leiomyomas, is usually the largest nodule; as such, it should be included in samples selected for freezing, together with any area where there is loss of interlacing fascicular pattern (Fig. 5.26).

Interpretation and Differential Diagnostic Considerations

Leiomyosarcoma and Other Smooth Muscle Neoplasms

Smooth muscle tumors are the most common benign and malignant mesenchymal neoplasms of the uterine corpus. Several variants and unusual growth patterns of these tumors have been reported. The diagnosis of frankly malignant or benign smooth muscle tumors is usually not problematic. However, many of these neoplasms have unusual characteristics or intermediate morphologic features that

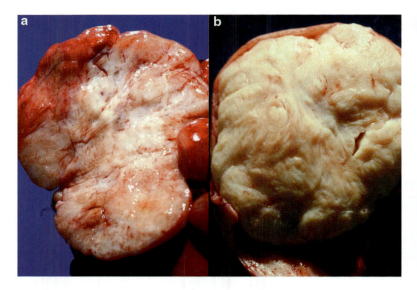

FIGURE 5.27 Leiomyosarcoma versus leiomyoma: (a) The cut surface of the large mass in Fig. 5.26 shows a homogeneous "fish-flesh" appearance and it lacks grossly visible fascicular pattern. (b) Cut surface of a leiomyoma showing a well-defined margin that separates the neoplasm from the surrounding myometrium. Interlacing fascicles of *yellowish-pink* muscle tissue and white fibrous tissue are evident. The fascicular pattern, however, can be lacking as a result of degenerative changes or necrosis in a benign leiomyoma. From Ramzy I. Essentials of gynecologic and obstetric pathology. 1983. Used with permission.

are difficult to classify, especially at time of frozen section. If there is any unusual pattern or histologic feature, the temporary diagnoses of smooth muscle tumor of uncertain malignant potential (STUMP) is rendered and the definite diagnosis deferred until permanent sections when extensive sampling with accurate mitotic counts and evaluation of other histologic parameters can be performed.
Worrisome features in which diagnosis of smooth muscle tumor of uncertain malignant potential (STUMP) is considered include presence of necrosis, significant cytologic atypia, and increased mitotic activity. Smooth muscle tumors with myxoid or epithelioid features with more than 2 mitosis/10 HPFs or atypia should also be considered as tumors of uncertain malignant potential.

In leiomyomas, the classic gross and microscopic appearance of interlacing fascicles of smooth muscle and fibrous tissue is helpful and usually easy to identify, in contrast to the homogeneous fish-flesh appearance of leiomyosarcoma (Fig. 5.27). Benign smooth

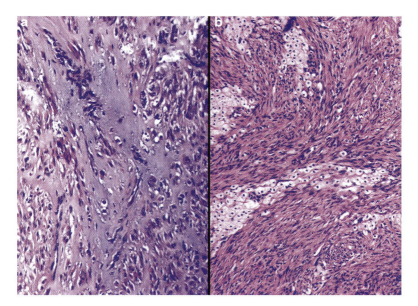

FIGURE 5.28 Variants of leiomyoma: (**a**) Myxoid change with no geographic pattern of necrosis. The degenerative changes can induce bizarre-shaped nuclei, but in such cases, mitotic figures are exceptionally rare and there is poor preservation of nuclear detail that results in blurring of the chromatin pattern (H&E, medium power). (**b**) Leiomyoma with clear cells. Nests of cells with clear cytoplasm and bland central nuclei are seen within the muscle bundles. Such a pattern is not a common feature of leiomyomas and should not be interpreted as nests of malignant clear epithelial cells (H&E, medium power).

muscle neoplasms can also manifest a variety of morphologic patterns, some of which are difficult to evaluate by frozen sections. The variants include cellular, myxoid, atypical, symplastic, and epithelioid leiomyomas (Figs. 5.28 and 5.29). Large lipoleiomyomas with mature adipose tissue elements may be occasionally encountered, as previously illustrated in Fig. 5.1. The key differentiating histologic criteria of some variants are summarized in Table 5.4.

The most critical differential diagnosis of leiomyoma is from leiomyosarcoma, particularly when there are degenerative changes in the tumor. Myxoid leiomyoma has a well-defined border that separates it from the surrounding myometrium, while myxoid leiomyosarcoma has an ill-defined invasive border, significant cytologic atypia, and tumor cell necrosis (Fig. 5.30). Necrosis can

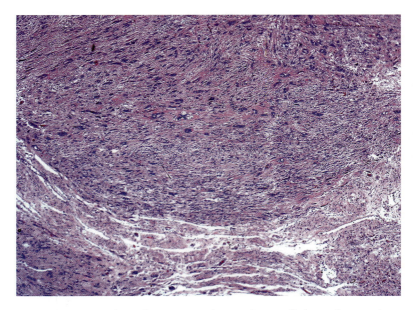

FIGURE 5.29 Symplastic leiomyoma: The neoplastic cells have pleomorphic, occasionally bizarre, nuclei. Unlike leiomyosarcoma, the change is focal and separated by pale collagen bands, rather than diffusely cellular. Although the nuclei are hyperchromatic, they show karyorrhexis and lack active mitosis (H&E, medium power).

TABLE 5.4 Key differentiating histologic features of smooth muscle neoplasms.

	Cellularity	Atypia	MF/10 HPF	Cell necrosis
Cellular	Cellular	None	4 or less	Absent
Symplastic	Normal	Bizarre cells	4 or less	Absent
Mitotically active	Variable	Minimal	>5 and <20	Absent or infarct type
Leiomyosarcoma	Cellular	Moderate/ high	10 or more	Present

be encountered in leiomyomas as a result of ischemic infarct, or in association with pregnancy (Fig. 5.31). In addition, coagulative tumor necrosis can be encountered as a result of previous therapy such as embolization or thermal ablation. The necrotic area is

UTERINE BODY 137

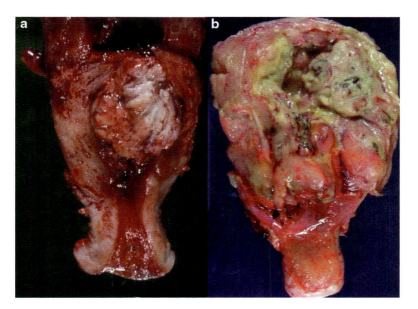

FIGURE 5.30 Myxoid leiomyoma and leiomyosarcoma: (**a**) This large leiomyoma shows myxoid change. The tumor is well defined, but has ulcerated and caused uterine bleeding and discharge. (**b**) Leiomyosarcoma showing myxoid change. Note the ill-defined borders and the invasive nature of the peripheral part of the tumor into the remainder of the myometrium.

well defined and maintains a ghost-like pattern of necrotic muscle bundles, unlike the geographic or ill-defined areas with individual tumor cell necrosis characteristic of leiomyosarcomas.

Accurate mitotic counts are often necessary for a definitive diagnosis and assessing the potential for aggressive behavior. Unfortunately, artifacts, including apoptosis, can simulate mitotic figures. In addition, benign smooth muscle tumors may be mitotically active, and unless there is significant atypia away from areas of necrosis, the differentiation of leiomyomas from leiomyosarcomas can be very difficult (Figs. 5.32 and 5.33). True vascular invasion supports the diagnosis of leiomyosarcoma. Leiomyomas often have abundant vascular channels between muscle bundles, but the neoplastic tissue is not seen within the lumen of these vessels, as is the case of leiomyosarcoma. Another entity that enters into the differential diagnosis is intravenous leiomyomatosis, characterized by cords of neoplastic

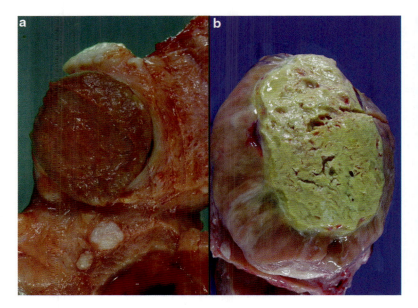

FIGURE 5.31 Leiomyomas with necrosis: (**a**) Leiomyoma showing the effect of ischemia. The *beefy red color* of the infarct is evident. (**b**) Smooth muscle tumor with necrosis. Although there is marked similarity to the tumor in Fig. 5.31a, malignancy could not be excluded despite extensive sampling, and the neoplasm was classified as smooth muscle tumor of uncertain malignant potential (STUMP).

smooth muscle cells within vascular channels. These neoplastic cells, however, have bland nuclei, low mitotic rate and they lack evidence of necrosis (Fig. 5.34).

Epithelioid Smooth Muscle Tumor

This variant of leiomyoma is characterized by at least 50% of tumor cells with polygonal or round epithelial-like morphology. Benign epithelioid leiomyomas may show poorly defined margins and a fleshy texture that raise the concern for a sarcoma. Microscopically, the cells have clear or eosinophilic cytoplasm and central round or oval nuclei (Fig. 5.35). Epithelioid leiomyomas have mild cytologic atypia, low mitotic rate (<3 mitosis/10 HPFs), and no tumor cell necrosis. The epithelioid cells are intermixed with the classic spindle cell bundles in about half the cases. The presence of nuclear atypia and increased (>5/10 HPFs) mitotic figures or geographic tumor

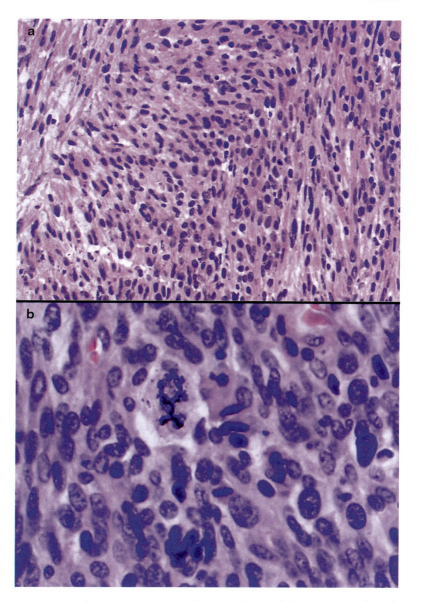

FIGURE 5.32 Leiomyosarcoma: **(a)** The cellularity of this neoplasm should raise the suspicion for malignancy, although identifying mitotic figures may not be easy in thick frozen sections. **(b)** In high-grade tumors, however, mitotic figures are easy to identify and establish the malignant nature of the tumor (H&E, a- medium power, b- high power).

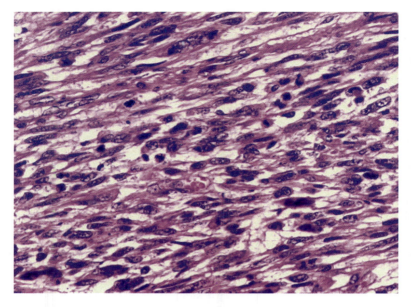

FIGURE 5.33 Leiomyosarcoma, showing bundles of spindled cells with abundant eosinophilic cytoplasm, nuclear pleomorphism associated with several mitotic figures and occasional multinucleation. Mitotic count should be performed only on permanent sections and apoptotic nuclei should be excluded from the count (H&E, medium power).

necrosis is diagnostic of epithelioid leiomyosarcoma. Epithelioid smooth muscle tumors are immunoreactive to vimentin, desmin, SMA, and can express cytokeratin. Lack of glandular differentiation and expression of smooth muscle markers differentiates these tumors from an undifferentiated carcinoma. Melanoma, perivascular epithelioid cell tumor (PEComa), and trophoblastic tumors should also be ruled out by negative staining of the smooth muscle tumor with HMB-45, S-100, and hPL.

Endometrial Stromal Sarcoma

These tumors account for 15% of uterine sarcomas and can be low grade endometrial stromal sarcoma or high grade undifferentiated sarcoma.

Low-grade endometrial stromal sarcoma produces nodular or diffuse thickening of the uterine wall, which may include the cervix (Fig. 5.36). The myometrium reveals raised islands of pink to tan

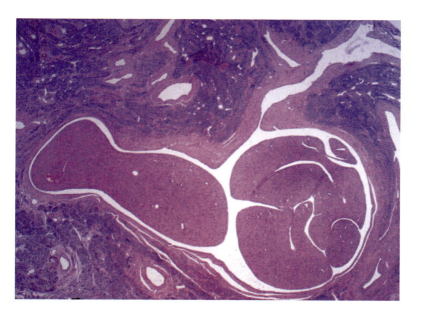

FIGURE 5.34 Intravenous leiomyomatosis: Cords of smooth muscle cells extend as finger-like structures within vascular channels. In other areas, the smooth muscle was attached to the wall, suggesting its origin from the wall of the vein, rather than from the myometrium. Despite its tendency to vascular spread, the neoplastic cells show no cytologic or nuclear features of malignancy (H&E, low power).

soft tissue, and areas of necrosis or hemorrhage may be present. The uterine cavity may be distended by a bulky polypoid mass that is covered by smooth intact endometrium, unlike the rough surface of polypoid adenocarcinoma. Low-grade endometrial stromal sarcomas have a propensity for vascular spread, with a third of the patients showing evidence of extrauterine pelvic spread at the time of surgery. The parametrial veins and lymphatics often contain "wormlike" cords or plugs of tumor (Figs. 5.37 and 5.38). Histologically, the tumor cells are uniform spindled or oval, with scant cytoplasm and may form morules around blood vessels, reminiscent of the spiral arterioles of the proliferative endometrium. Nuclear pleomorphism is minimal, if any, and mitotic figures are infrequent.

Endometrial stromal sarcomas should be differentiated from adenosarcoma, stromal nodule, cellular smooth muscle

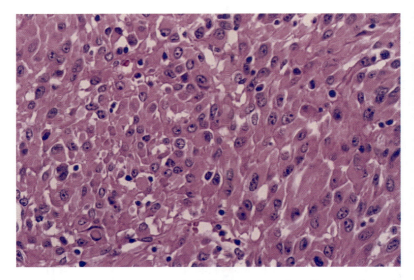

FIGURE 5.35 Leiomyosarcoma, epithelioid variant: The cells are polygonal rather than spindled, and they have abundant eosinophilic cytoplasm. The nuclei are centrally located and bland. Unlike adenocarcinomas, the neoplastic cells lack gland formations and they react to smooth muscle markers (H&E, medium power).

neoplasms, adenomyosis, and the rare sex cord-like uterine tumors. Adenosarcoma has abundant glands, and these are surrounded by sarcomatous stromal cells. It rarely involves the myometrium or shows the vascular pattern of spread characteristic of stromal sarcoma. Endometrial stromal nodules consist of cells identical to those of LGESS, but are well circumscribed and usually limited to the endometrium (Fig. 5.39). Occasionally, foci of adenomyosis may have scant glands, but the presence of foci with glands and smooth muscle in other areas or in deeper cuts in the frozen section block, as well as the lack of vascular invasion favor the diagnosis of adenomyosis. Cellular smooth muscle neoplasms have been discussed previously, but occasionally they may involve vascular channels simulating LGESS. Sex cord-like uterine tumors consist almost exclusively of cells showing sex cord-like differentiation, unlike the rare focus encountered in LGESS.

Undifferentiated (high-grade) endometrial sarcomas tend to be bulky, show areas of necrosis and hemorrhage, often with partially intact endometrial surface. There is destructive myometrial

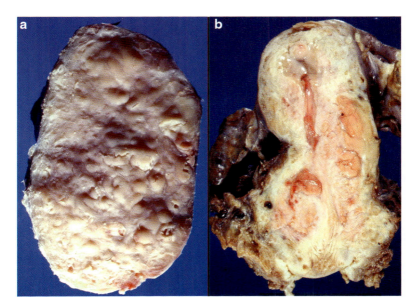

FIGURE 5.36 Endometrial stromal sarcoma, gross: (**a**) This nodule, from a 28-year-old patient who desired fertility preservation, was initially submitted as leiomyoma. The myometrium has raised islands of soft *pink* to tan areas of stroma. Following the frozen section report, a hysterectomy was performed. (**b**) The hysterectomy specimen revealed raised islands of tumor tissue involving the uterine corpus and cervix. The tumor was also seen within some of the parametrial veins.

invasion but the tumor lacks the wormlike intravascular permeation of LGESS. Microscopically, there is increased cellularity, with the neoplastic cells showing prominent nuclear atypia, multinucleated giant cells, and abundant mitotic figures (10–20/HPF) (Fig. 5.40). Evidence of endometrial stromal differentiation is lacking, and some pathologists prefer the term poorly differentiated or high-grade uterine sarcoma. The diagnosis of a high-grade sarcoma is usually an easy one to establish by frozen section. Sampling of multiple areas for permanent sections is necessary, in order to exclude the presence of other homologous or heterologous elements in the tumor.

Carcinosarcoma (Malignant Mixed Müllerian Tumor)
These highly malignant neoplasms account for almost half of the uterine sarcomas. Carcinosarcomas are bulky neoplasms that

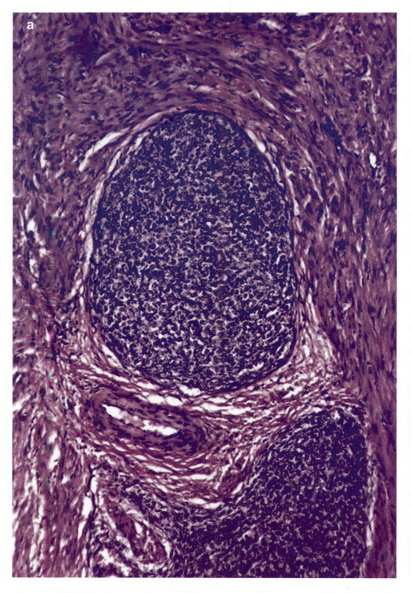

FIGURE 5.37 Endometrial stromal sarcoma, low grade: (**a**) Islands of endometrial stroma within myometrial tissue spaces, lymphatics, or blood vessels (H&E, low power). (**b**) The neoplastic cells are uniform, with bland nuclei and scant cytoplasm similar to normal endometrial stromal cells (H&E, medium power). (**c**) Small blood vessels, reminiscent of spiral arterioles may be seen, and only a few mitotic figures (usually <3 per 10 HPF) are encountered (H&E, medium power).

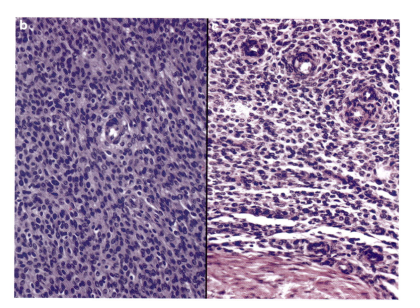

Figure 5.37 (continued)

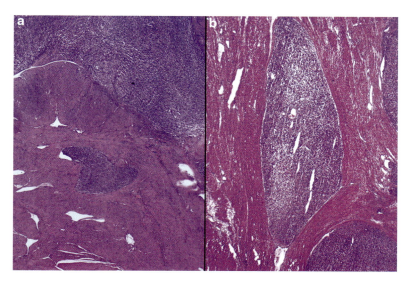

Figure 5.38 Leiomyosarcoma simulating stromal sarcoma: (**a**) Plugs of leiomyosarcoma within lymphatics may simulate low-grade endometrial stromal sarcoma. The cytoplasm is usually more abundant and eosinophilic than that of stromal sarcoma (H&E, low power). (**b**) Stromal sarcoma demonstrates spiral arteriole-like vessels unlike the leiomyosarcoma (H&E, low power).

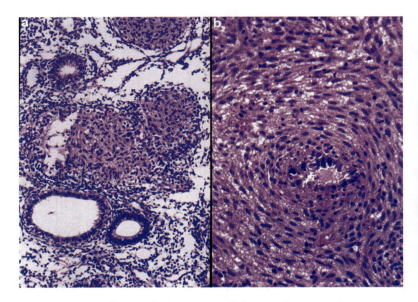

FIGURE 5.39 Differential diagnosis of low-grade stromal sarcoma: (**a**) Endometrial stromal nodules are small, often microscopic, nests of stromal cells within the endometrium and spare the myometrium. The cells are uniform, with a low mitotic count (usually less than 3/10HPF) (H&E, low power). (**b**) Prolonged administration of progestational agents can induce marked stromal response. The cells are plump, but they form concentric bundles around small endometrial glands that show evidence of nuclear degeneration and homogenization of chromatin (H&E, medium power).

distend the endometrial cavity deeply, invade the myometrium, and frequently present at an advanced stage with extrauterine involvement. Hemorrhage and necrosis are commonly present (Fig. 5.41). Histologically, several malignant heterologous or homologous epithelial and stromal components are encountered. Common epithelial elements include endometrioid, serous and, less frequently, mucinous, squamous, or clear-cell differentiation (Fig. 5.42). Mesenchymal elements include smooth muscle, endometrial stroma, or undifferentiated spindle cell sarcoma. Heterologous elements include differentiation along cartilaginous, osseous, skeletal muscle, and/or adipose tissue lines (Fig. 5.43).

Identification of various epithelial and mesenchymal elements helps to differentiate MMMT from leiomyosarcomas endometrial stromal sarcomas and adenosarcoma. However, if only one element is seen at the time of frozen section, it is prudent to classify

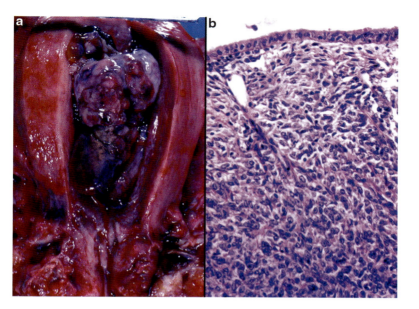

FIGURE 5.40 Endometrial stromal sarcoma, high grade (undifferentiated endometrial sarcoma): (**a**) A bulky hemorrhagic tumor distends the uterine cavity. There is surface ulceration (H&E, medium power). (**b**) Endometrial stromal cells showing nuclear pleomorphism and hyperchromasia. Mitosis is often above 10/10 HPF. The cytoplasm is amphophilic. Note the absence of any endometrial gland component. In several fields, the tumor cells show little resemblance to stromal cells, and differential diagnosis from other undifferentiated sarcomas may be difficult (H&E, medium power). From Ramzy I. Essentials of gynecologic and obstetric pathology. Norwalk: Appleton Century Crofts; 1983. p. 201. Used with permission.

the lesion as high-grade neoplasm or sarcoma, and defer final classification until additional samples are procured for permanent sections, and select battery of immunostains used to identify other components, if necessary. Endometrioid carcinomas rarely have heterologous elements, but these are usually small foci of mature tissues without any sarcomatous features. The presence of heterologous elements and immunoreactivity of the sarcomatous component to vimentin, smooth muscle actin, as well as epithelial markers differentiates MMMT from sarcomatoid endometrioid carcinoma. Rarely, the tumor consists of malignant glands and a bland fibrous stroma, and such cases have been classified as carcinofibroma by WHO criteria (Fig. 5.44).

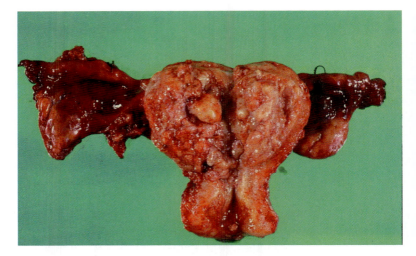

FIGURE 5.41 Carcinosarcoma: A large polymorphous and friable tumor distends the uterine cavity, infiltrating the entire thickness of myometrium and part of the cervix.

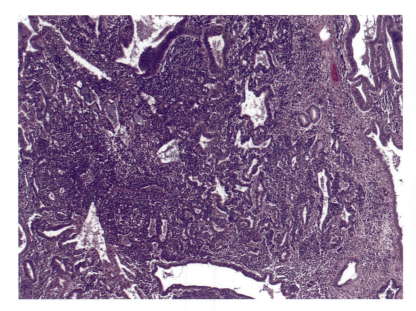

FIGURE 5.42 Carcinosarcoma: There is a wide variety of homologous and heterologous epithelial as well as connective tissues (H&E low power).

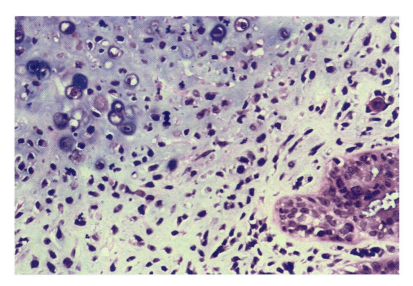

FIGURE 5.43 Carcinosarcoma: Malignant cartilage, undifferentiated mesenchyme, glands, and an isolated keratinized cell are components of this heterologous tumor (H&E, medium power). From Ramzy I. Essentials of gynecologic and obstetric pathology. Norwalk: Appleton Century Crofts; 1983. p. 204. Used with permission.

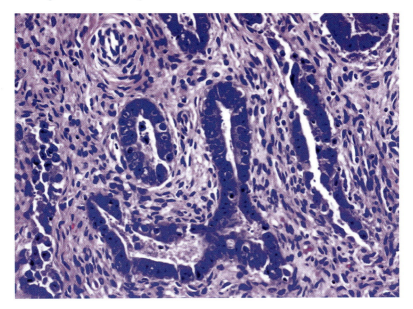

FIGURE 5.44 "Carcinofibroma": The tumor consists of malignant glands in an apparently benign fibrous tissue background. Many authors classify this as a variant of carcinosarcoma (H&E, high power).

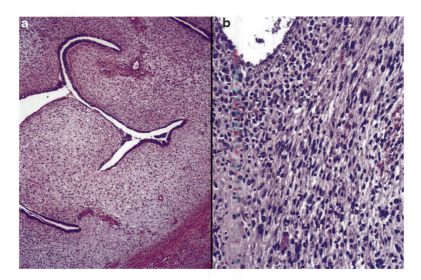

FIGURE 5.45 Adenosarcoma: (**a**) Malignant stromal cells incorporating clefts that are lined by uniform benign epithelium (H&E, low power). (**b**) At higher magnification, the stromal cells show nuclear pleomorphism and hyperchromasia. The gland is lined by a single layer of uniform epithelial cells (H&E, medium power).

Adenosarcoma

Most adenosarcomas present as endometrial polypoid lesions originating from the endometrium, and occasionally from the cervix. They have a spongy or cystic cut surface and are usually limited to the mucosa. The histologic features are similar to those of endometrial stromal sarcoma, except for the presence of Müllerian glands as integral components throughout the tumor. These glands are mostly endometrioid, but endocervical, clear-cell and ciliated epithelia may also be encountered (Fig. 5.45). Although the glands are cytologically bland, they can be cystic, hyperplastic, or atypical. The stroma shows condensation near the glands, where mitotic figures can be readily identified (~4/10 HPF). Heterologous elements are uncommon. Adenosarcoma rarely invades the underlying myometrium. It should be differentiated from a few neoplasms and non-neoplastic polypoid masses. Cellular endometrial polyps, atypical polypoid adenomyoma, and Müllerian adenofibromas lack the characteristic periglandular cuffing, cytologic atypia, and mitotic activity of the malignant stroma. In endometrial stromal sarcoma, the epithelial elements are sparse and encountered at the edge of the tumor (see above). In MMMT, the epithelial elements manifest malignant features.

RECOMMENDED READING

Abeler VM, Nenodovic M. Diagnostic immunohistochemistry in uterine sarcomas: A study of 397 cases. Internat J Gynecol Pathol. 2011;30:336–43.

Altintas A, Cosar E, Vardar MA, et al. Intraoperative assessment of depth of myometrial invasion in endometrial carcinoma. Eur J Gynaecol Oncol. 1999;20:329–31.

Atad J, Weill S, Ben-David Y, et al. Intraoperative frozen section examination of myometrial invasion depth in patients with endometrial carcinoma. Int J Gynecol Cancer. 1994;4:352–5.

Attard MS, Coutts M, Devaja O, et al. Accuracy of frozen section diagnosis at surgery in pre-malignant and malignant lesions of the endometrium. Eur J Gynaecol Oncol. 2008;29:435–40.

Barakat RR, Bevers MW, Gershenson DM, Hoskins WH, editors. MD Anderson Cancer Center and Memorial Sloan-Kettering Cancer Center Handbook of gynecologic oncology. 2nd ed. London: Martin Dunitz; 2002.

Berek JS, Hacker NF, editors. Berek & Hacker's practical gynecologic oncology. 5th ed. Philadelphia, PA: Lippincott Williams & Wilkins; 2009.

Bjornsson BL, Nelson BE, Reale FR, Rose PG. Accuracy of frozen section for lymph node metastasis in patients undergoing radical hysterectomy for carcinoma of the cervix. Gynecol Oncol. 1993;51:50–3.

Boronow RC, Morrow CP, Creasman WT, et al. Surgical staging in endometrial cancer: clinical-pathologic findings of a prospective study. Obstet Gynecol. 1984;63:825–32.

Creasman WT, Morrow CP, Bundy BN, et al. Surgical pathologic spread of endometrial cancer, a gynecologic oncology group study. Cancer. 1987;60:2035–41.

Crum CP, Lee KR, editors. Diagnostic gynecologic and obstetric pathology. Philadelphia, PA: Elsevier Saunders; 2006.

Daniel AG, Peters 3rd WA. Accuracy of office and operating room curettage in the grading of endometrial carcinoma. Obstet Gynecol. 1988;71:612–4.

DiSaia PJ, Creasman WT. Clinical gynecologic oncology. 7th ed. Philadelphia, PA: Mosby-Elsevier; 2007.

Fanfani F, Ludovisi M, Zannoni GF, et al. Frozen section examination of pelvic lymph nodes in endometrial and cervical cancer: accuracy in patients submitted to neoadjuvant treatments. Gynecol Oncol. 2004;94:779–84.

Fishman A et al. The value of transvaginal sonography in the preoperative assessment of myometrial invasion in high and low grade endometrial cancer and in comparison to frozen section in grade 1 disease. Eur J Gynaecol Oncol. 2000;21:128–30.

Forde GK, Carlson JW, Downey GO, et al. A quality process study of lymph node evaluation in endometrial cancer. Internat J Gynecol Pathol. 2011;30:335–9.

Goff BA, Rice LW. Assessment of depth of myometrial invasion in endometrial adenocarcinoma. Gynecol Oncol. 1990;38:46–8.

Hasenburg A et al. Evaluation of lymph nodes in squamous cell carcinoma of the cervix: touch imprint cytology versus frozen section histology. Int J Gynecol Cancer. 1999;9:337–41.

Hoskins W, Perez CA, Young RC. Principles and practice of gynecologic oncology. 3rd ed. Philadelphia, PA: Lippincott William & Wilkins; 2000.

Indermaur M, Shoup B, Tebes S, et al. The accuracy of frozen pathology at time of hysterectomy in patients with complex atypical hyperplasia on preoperative biopsy. Residents' papers. Am J Obstet Gynecol. 2007;196:e40–2.

Kir G, Kir M, Cetiner H, et al. Diagnostic problems on frozen section examination of myometrial invasion in patients with endometrial carcinoma with special emphasis on the pitfalls of deep adenomyosis with carcinomatous involvement. Eur J Gynaecol Oncol. 2004;25:211–4.

Korczynski J, Jesionek-Kupnicka D, Gottwald L, et al. Comparison of FIGO 1989 and 2009 recommendations on staging of endometrial carcinoma. Pathologic analysis and cervical status in 123 consecutive cases. Internat J Gynecol Pathol. 2011;30:328–34.

Kucera E, Kainz RC, Sliutz G, et al. Accuracy of intraoperative frozen section diagnosis in stage I endometrial adenocarcinoma. Gynecol Obstet Invest. 2000;49:62–6.

Lopez-Garcia MA, Palacios J. Pathologic and molecular features of uterine carcinosarcomas. Semin Diagn Pathol 2010;27:274–86.

Mills SE. Decidua and squamous metaplasia in abdominopelvic lymph nodes. Int J Gynecol Pathol. 1983;2:209–15.

Noriaki S, Chikara S, Naoki T, et al. Incidence and distribution pattern of pelvic and paraaortic lymph node metastasis in patients with Stage IB, IIA and IIB cervical carcinoma treated with radical hysterectomy. Cancer. 1999;85:1547–54.

Noumoff JS, Menzin A, Mikuta J, et al. The ability to evaluate prognostic variables on frozen section in hysterectomies performed for endometrial carcinoma. Gynecol Oncol. 1991;42:202–8.

Nucci MR, Oliva E. Gynecologic pathology. London: Elsevier Churchill Livingstone; 2009 (Volume in the series foundations in diagnostic pathology).

Robboy SJ, Anderson MC, Russell P. Pathology of the female reproductive tract. London: Churchill Livingstone; 2002.

Shim JU, Rose PG, Reale FR, et al. Accuracy of frozen section diagnosis at surgery in clinical stage I and II endometrial carcinoma. Am J Obstet Gynecol. 1992;166:1335–8.

Takeshima N, Hirai Y, Hasumi K. Prognostic validity of neoplastic cells with notable nuclear atypia in endometrial cancer. Obstet Gynecol. 1998;92:119–23.

Wu DC, Hirschowitz S, Nararajan S. Ectopic decidua of pelvic lymph nodes. Arch Pathol Lab Med. 2005;129:117–20.

Chapter 6
Ovary and Fallopian Tube

Ovarian cancer is the fourth most frequent cause of cancer death in women. It accounts for 5% of all cancer deaths, with a mortality rate that exceeds the combined rates of cervical and endometrial carcinoma. Early detection is elusive as many cases present with nonspecific symptoms and are identified late in the course of the disease. A wide variety of non-neoplastic functional, inflammatory lesions of the ovary, the tube, and the broad ligament also result in the development of adnexal masses. Surgical exploration is indicated in many of these cases in order to clarify the nature of the lesions and manage the disease (Table 6.1). Gross and frozen section consultations are often needed to establish the neoplastic nature of an ovarian mass and help in differentiating benign tumors from borderline or malignant ones. Although a detailed discussion of the pathology of ovarian tumors is beyond the scope of this text, consideration of the different types is important, since handling such specimens should be tailored to the suspected tumor type, size, and the clinical presentation, with an emphasis on answering questions that will have an impact on the type and extent of surgery. Interpretation by frozen sections is also utilized to determine the presence of peritoneal spread and differentiation of primary from metastatic malignancies (Table 6.2). The status of the pelvic lymph nodes plays only a minor role in the immediate intraoperative decision-making in the case of ovarian lesions; thus, lymph node sampling for frozen section consultation is not routinely requested. Rarely, a biopsy is performed in cases of ovarian failure, and such cases require consultation with the surgeon prior to the procedure, to ensure proper handling of the specimen.

TABLE 6.1 Adnexal mass: indications for surgery.

Ovarian cystic structure >5 cm followed 6–8 weeks without regression
Solid ovarian lesion
Ovarian lesion with papillary vegetations on the cyst wall
Adnexal mass >10 cm in diameter
Ascites
Palpable adnexal mass in a premenarchal or postmenopausal patient
Suspicion of torsion or rupture
Biopsy for ovarian failure

Modified from DiSaia PJ, Creasman WT. Clinical gynecologic oncology. 7th ed. Philadelphia, PA: Moby-Elsevier; 2007. Used with permission.

TABLE 6.2 Questions to be answered by intraoperative consults in adnexal masses.

Establishing the diagnosis of neoplasia
Establishing the diagnosis of malignancy
Degree of malignancy if present, borderline versus frankly malignant
Type of neoplasm: primary versus metastatic
Type and subtype of primary neoplasm: epithelial, sex cord/stromal, or germ cell
Nature of peritoneal nodules
Nature of adhesions

GENERAL CONSIDERATIONS

Benign tumors are commonly smooth-walled, cystic, mobile, unilateral, and smaller than 8 cm in diameter. Malignant tumors, in contrast, are usually solid or semisolid, fixed, and associated with ascites or nodules in the cul de sac. The diagnostic accuracy of intraoperative consultation of ovarian lesions depends on the type of lesion, its size, and extent of sampling, among other factors, such as the experience of the pathologist. Frozen section consults have a sensitivity of 86%, specificity close to 100%, positive predictive value of 100%, and negative predictive value of 95% for malignancy. The overall diagnostic accuracy ranges from 87 to 96%. False negative and false positive diagnoses are most common in cases of large ovarian masses and in borderline tumors. In addition, difficulties in differentiating primary from metastatic ovarian tumors are well documented. Consults limited to gross examination only have a concordance rate of 94.7%, with the most common pitfall being the misinterpretation of a borderline cystic lesion, since the malignancy may be focal and require sampling of multiple areas of the tumor. Frozen sections should be performed in any case where

TABLE 6.3 Factors in assessing risk at time of intraoperative consultation.

Age
Menstrual history
Bilaterality
Size of tumor
Ultrasound characteristics of the mass
Any family history of breast or ovarian cancer (BRCA1 or BRCA2 status)
History of previous malignancy

TABLE 6.4 Most common ovarian neoplasms.

Cystic neoplasms	Solid neoplasms
Benign	Benign
Serous cystadenoma	Fibroma
Mucinous cystadenoma	Thecoma
Cystic teratoma	
Malignant	Malignant
Serous cystadenocarcinoma	Adenocarcinomas, primary
Mucinous cystadenocarcinoma	Adenocarcinomas, metastatic

malignancy is suspected clinically, thus minimizing the risk of undertreatment.

Careful preoperative consideration of factors such as age, menopausal status, and bilaterality helps determine the risks of malignant disease, and the surgeon must communicate to the pathologist all such pertinent clinical information and the cancer risk, to avoid false negative diagnosis (Table 6.3).

The patient's age helps in prioritizing the lesions to be considered in the differential diagnosis. In premenarchal and postmenopausal patients, an adnexal mass is considered highly abnormal and should be immediately investigated. Any enlargement of the ovaries in the postmenopausal age group is considered malignant until proven otherwise. Germ cell tumors are the most common ovarian neoplasms in the premenarchal age, while stromal, epithelial, and metastatic tumors are mostly seen in postmenopausal patients. For the reproductive age group, both benign and malignant tumors are included in the differential diagnosis, with the majority of these neoplasms being histologically benign. Table 6.4 lists the most commonly-encountered ovarian neoplasms.

OVARIAN AND TUBAL SPECIMENS

The adnexa are often resected in association with a hysterectomy for uterine pathologies, particularly in postmenopausal women. Except for a few situations, such as torsion or acute salpingooophoritis, the majority of these surgeries are elective. These only require gross examination of the ovary or tube at the time of surgery; a section of the tube and ovary, to include the hilum and cortex, is processed for permanent sections. Frozen sections are not performed unless an unexpected adnexal abnormality is encountered.

However, when the procedure is performed primarily because of an adnexal pathology, the type of specimen submitted to the laboratory depends on the indication for surgery, risk of malignancy, and other clinical considerations, such as history of previous neoplasms in the ovary, breast, or gastrointestinal tract. These specimens may be in the form of cystectomy, unilateral or bilateral resection of the ovaries and/or tubes, or biopsy of an adhesion/nodule. A biopsy of the ovary is performed when a lesion on the surface is encountered during surgery, to ensure its benign nature by frozen section examination, but rarely in the context of investigating a fertility problem.

Staging

Adequate staging of ovarian cancer is crucial since the survival of patients is directly correlated with tumor stage. After a rigorous staging laparotomy, many patients initially classified as having localized disease will be upstaged. In cases of borderline malignancy, surgeons often elect to "stage" the tumor with frozen section consultation; this avoids the need for a second operation if invasion is identified in the final report. If the borderline lesion is unilateral, a salpingooophorectomy with thorough examination of the contralateral ovary, peritoneal washings, and partial omentectomy are performed. If the lesions are bilateral, show surface involvement or peritoneal spread, as well as in frankly malignant tumors confined to the ovary or pelvis, a more radical surgery, including total abdominal hysterectomy, bilateral salpingooophorectomy, and thorough surgical staging is performed. The staging procedure includes collection of any free fluid or peritoneal washings, omentectomy, multiple biopsies of the peritoneum and diaphragm, as well as sampling of pelvic and paraaortic lymph nodes. A positive pleural fluid or fine needle aspirate of the supraclavicular lymph nodes can also be used to document a stage IV disease.

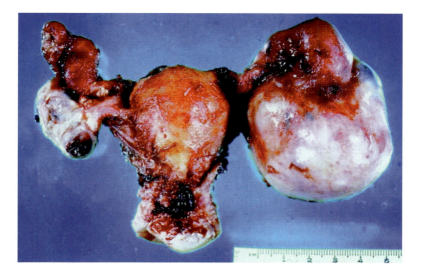

FIGURE 6.1 Salpingooophorectomy: The left fallopian tube is stretched over an ovarian neoplasm in a hysterectomy and bilateral salpingooophorectomy specimen.

OOPHORECTOMY AND SALPINGOOOPHORECTOMY

This is one of the most common types of ovarian samples submitted for intraoperative consultation. Resection of the ovary is usually associated with resection of the adjoining fallopian tube. Handling these specimens depends upon the size and type of lesion suspected, and addressing issues that have an immediate impact on the operative procedure. Open communication between the pathologist and the surgeon regarding any suspicious foci should help in selecting areas to be sampled.

Specimen Handling

Oophorectomies for cystic ovarian neoplasms and cystectomies are examined in a similar fashion. The external surface of the ovary and fallopian tube is examined for any areas of excrescences, nodularity, disruption, or adhesions (Fig. 6.1). If the lesion is cystic, the cyst is opened, and the quality and color of the fluid are documented. Cystic neoplasms can be unilocular or multilocular lesions. In general, unilocular cysts with smooth walls are benign. Any areas of thickening of the cyst wall, complex architecture, granularity, intraluminal or surface papillary projections, hemorrhage, or necrosis must be noted. If solid areas are encountered, the size of these areas should be documented, as well as their color noted.

Large tumors should be grossly examined thoroughly and multiple sections submitted, to increase sensitivity for focal borderline changes. Any residual ovarian tissue should be identified in the wall of large cysts. Surface adhesions or evidence of rupture should be noted, since it may indicate dissemination into the peritoneal cavity. The surface of the mass should be examined, and the specimen sliced at 1 cm intervals, starting with the most suspicious or solid areas, to avoid unnecessary delay in the intraoperative consult. Sampling should include papillae, solid components or thickened cyst wall, as well as areas closest to the capsule or surface. Since grossly necrotic or hemorrhagic areas often do not yield any recognizable diagnostic tissue, they should not be selected for freezing.

CYSTECTOMY

Clinical Background

Cysts are resected and submitted for consultation to determine their nature and subsequent planning of the surgery (Fig. 6.2). Cystectomies are usually performed for benign-appearing lesions,

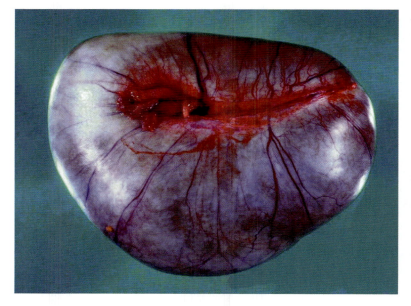

FIGURE 6.2 Simple cystectomy for a serous cystadenoma.

or in patients who wish to preserve fertility, particularly since many benign tumors, such as teratomas, occur during the third and fourth decades of life. Patients in this age group are also more likely to develop non-neoplastic cysts that require a conservative approach. Non-neoplastic cysts include functional cysts such as corpus luteal and follicular cysts, theca lutein cysts, pregnancy luteoma, polycystic ovaries, as well as endometriotic cysts.

Specimen Handling and Interpretation

Cysts should be submitted intact; their size and weight should be recorded before they are opened. The consistency of the content should be examined and some of the fluid can be preserved for additional tests, such as smear preparation, if necessary. The external surface is examined for any adhesions, excrescences and the capsule noted for any tears or infiltration by neoplastic tissue. As a general rule, approximately one section for every 1–2 cm diameter of the cyst is adequate for permanent sections. To conserve time during intraoperative consultation, however, the pathologist should select areas of papillary proliferations, thickening in the wall, or solid components for frozen section as previously discussed. A roll of the cyst wall or multiple strips can be placed in one block to maximize the sampling without increasing the time needed before a diagnosis is rendered.

OVARIAN BIOPSY

This is not a common method of sampling the ovary; most are biopsies of an incidental lesion encountered during surgery and submitted for frozen section consultation to ensure its benign nature. Occasionally, the ovary is sampled as part of the investigation of fertility problems. In such cases, a consult between the surgeon and the pathologist should be arranged prior to the procedure, to discuss the reason for the biopsy, the location, and size of the sample, and to ensure optimal handling and triaging of the fresh tissue. Wedge biopsies for polycystic ovarian disease are not usually submitted for intraoperative consultation (Fig. 6.3). Small biopsies should be oriented properly, fixed promptly, and submitted for processing as paraffin blocks. The operative consultation in such cases does not involve frozen sections for immediate interpretation of the biopsy, but the presence of hemorrhagic endometriotic foci, corpora lutea, or follicular cysts should be noted in the final report.

160   FROZEN SECTION LIBRARY

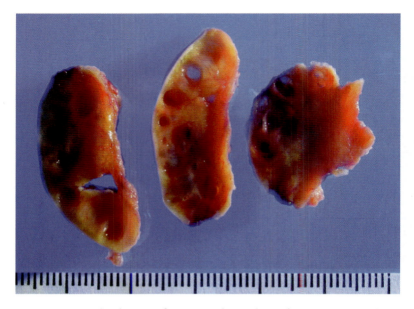

FIGURE 6.3 Wedge biopsy of ovaries: The wedges of ovarian tissue show multiple cysts and fibrous thickened ovarian capsules. The 25-year-old patient had amenorrhea and evidence of hirsutism associated with polycystic ovarian disease.

OMENTAL AND PERITONEAL BIOPSIES

Nodules discovered at the time of surgery on the omental surface, cul-de-sac, or intestinal serosa, are often submitted for frozen evaluation (Fig. 6.4). The result of such microscopic examination determines the course of action and the feasibility of a successful resection of a neoplasm. Examination of touch imprints can provide a quick and reliable alternative or a complimentary method to detect malignant cells in such specimens (Fig. 6.5).

LYMPH NODE SAMPLING

Pelvic and abdominal lymph nodes may be a part of the surgical procedure when an ovarian cancer is suspected, and these samples can be submitted for frozen section evaluation. Trimming the adipose tissue intimately related to the node helps in minimizing the technical difficulty in cutting thin and complete sections, in view of the difficulty in freezing fat. The subcapsular sinuses should be carefully examined for microscopic deposits. The pathologist must

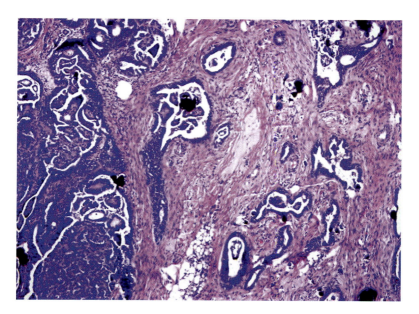

FIGURE 6.4 Omental biopsy: The peritoneal nodule was biopsied during resection of a borderline serous tumor of the ovary. The features are those of a peritoneal implant, discussed later (H&E, medium power).

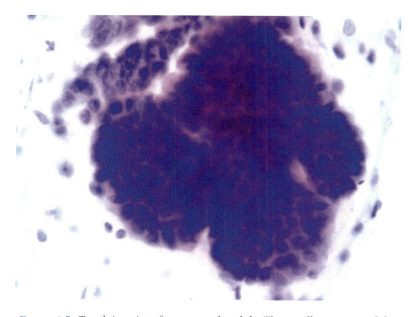

FIGURE 6.5 Touch imprint of an omental nodule. The papillary nature of the neoplasm is evident (Papanicolaou stain, high power).

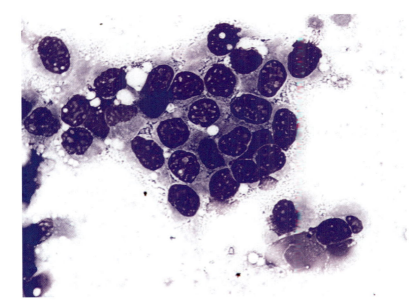

FIGURE 6.6 Gutter lavage showing a cluster of malignant cells from a serous papillary carcinoma of ovary (Air-dryed, Diff-Quik, high power, oil).

consider cytologic atypia and necrosis due to preoperative chemotherapy given in some ovarian cancer cases that may lead to an inaccurate interpretation. In young patients, especially in pregnant patients, ectopic decidua may form nodules on the ovarian surface, peritoneum or lymph nodes that may be misinterpreted as metastatic foci of squamous cell carcinoma.

PELVIC, PERITONEAL AND GUTTER LAVAGES
These cytologic specimens are routinely submitted from ovarian malignancies since they provide valuable information regarding staging and outcome. Rapid staining using a Romanowsky stain such as Diff-Quik may be helpful if malignant cells are present in large numbers (Fig. 6.6). However, any proper examination requires time for processing and, therefore, immediate evaluation in a timely fashion is usually not feasible during the surgical procedure.

INTERPRETATION AND DIFFERENTIAL DIAGNOSIS IN ADNEXAL LESIONS
The interpretation and differential diagnostic issues encountered in the frozen section laboratory are governed by the wide variety of neoplasms and non-neoplastic cysts that involve the ovary. The

non-neoplastic spectrum encompasses functional lesions and cysts, inflammatory masses, and endometriotic lesions. The neoplasms include benign, borderline, and frankly malignant tumors of epithelial, sex cord/stromal, germ cell, and nonspecific tumors of unknown histogenesis. Some non-gynecologic malignancies, such as breast and gastrointestinal cancers, have a predilection for metastasis to the ovaries and add to the list of potential sources that should be considered in the differential diagnosis of adnexal masses.

Gross diagnosis of cystic ovarian masses should be avoided in high risk patients, such as patients with elevated CA125 or in known mutation carrier patients. In cystectomy cases where a borderline lesion is suspected, it is recommended to report these lesions as "at least borderline tumor" or "rule out borderline tumor." In these cases, the surgeon may extend the surgery to perform a total oophorectomy and omentectomy. Extensive necrosis, hemorrhage, or inflammation can also obscure the frozen section examination, thus limiting the diagnostic ability. In cases of borderline malignancy, the cyst is usually lined, at least in part, by lush papillary projections. Extensive sampling of such areas is required to rule out invasion. If invasion is not clearly seen on the frozen section, the lesion may be classified as borderline, with a clear statement and understanding that invasive carcinoma can be ruled out only after more extensive sampling is performed on permanent sections.

NON-NEOPLASTIC LESIONS

Several non-neoplastic tumor-like conditions that should be considered in the differential diagnosis of ovarian neoplasms by frozen section are listed in Table 6.5.

Endometriotic cysts, oophoritis, stromal hyperplasia, and hyperthecosis, as well as massive ovarian edema can be clinically

TABLE 6.5 Non-neoplastic lesions presenting as adnexal masses.

Functional cysts: follicular, theca lutein, luteal
Luteoma of pregnancy
Salpingooophoritis and tuboovarian abscess: acute and chronic
Endometriosis
Torsion
Ectopic pregnancy
Stromal hyperplasia
Hyperthecosis
Leydig cell hyperplasia
Massive ovarian edema

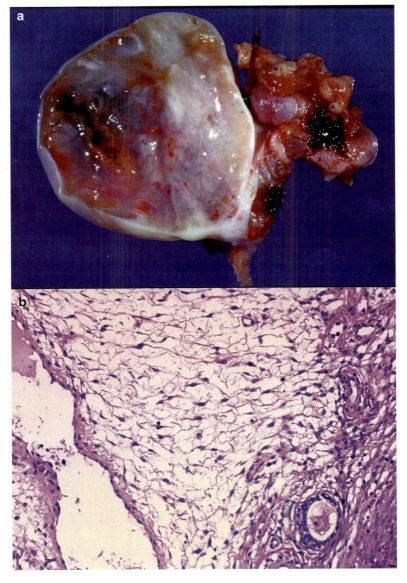

FIGURE 6.7 Massive edema of the ovary: (**a**) The patient presented with an adnexal mass. The enlarged ovary had a soft consistency and shining surface (H&E, medium power). (**b**) Ovarian stromal cells are separated by accumulation of fluid. Presence of follicles differentiates this from a neoplasm of the fibrothecoma group (H&E, medium power).

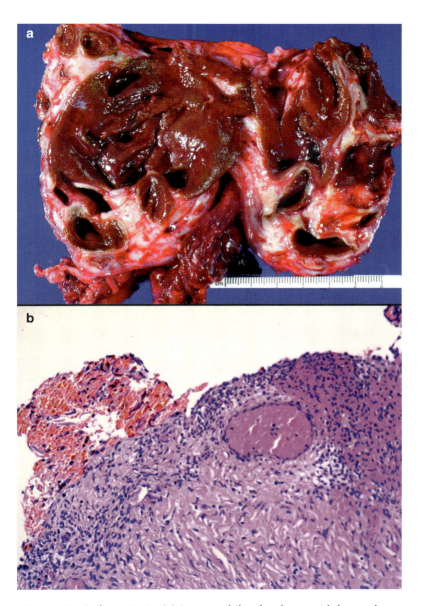

FIGURE 6.8 Endometriosis: (**a**) Large multiloculated cyst with hemorrhage (chocolate cyst), fibrosis of the ovarian tissue. The outer surface had fibrous adhesions that involved the pelvic peritoneum (H&E, medium power). (**b**) Endometrial glands and stroma may be scant and overshadowed by hemorrhage and fibrosis. Several sections may be needed before a viable diagnostic area is identified. Poor preservation of nuclear and cytoplasmic features helps in differentiating atypical degenerating cells lining the cyst from malignant epithelium (H&E, medium power).

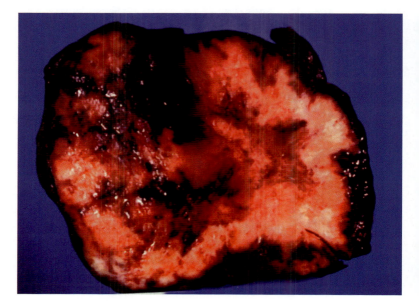

FIGURE 6.9 Ovarian torsion: The ovary is hemorrhagic and must be carefully examined to determine the cause of the torsion, since it may be due to the presence of a cyst or neoplasm. In this case, torsion was the result of a benign transitional cell neoplasm (Brenner) which became infarcted.

worrisome, since they present as adnexal masses at the time of laparoscopy or gynecologic examination. Luteomas of pregnancy, multiple theca-lutein cysts, solitary follicular cysts of pregnancy, and Leydig cell hyperplasia tend to spontaneously involute without the need for surgery, while others, such as ruptured ectopic pregnancy and ovarian torsion require urgent exploration. Clinical features, history, imaging studies, and gross intraoperative consultations clarify the nature of many cases. However, frozen section plays an important role in establishing the diagnosis in problematic cases. Features that help differentiating these from neoplasms are illustrated and detailed in Figs. 6.7–6.10.

SURFACE EPITHELIAL TUMORS

Epithelial neoplasms are the most commonly encountered forms of ovarian tumors. They may show serous, mucinous, endometrioid, clear cell, or transitional cell differentiation, with serous adenocarcinoma being the single most common malignancy, and its benign counterpart the most common benign ovarian neoplasm

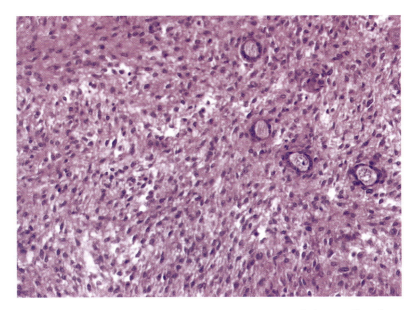

FIGURE 6.10 Thecomatosis: The hyperplastic luteinized theca cells, often seen in both ovaries, are diffusely arranged and encompass follicles or corpora albicantia, in contrast to forming a well circumscribed mass in theca cell tumors (H&E, medium power).

(Tables 6.6 and 6.7). All epithelial tumors often show transition from benign to borderline to malignant areas, thus facilitating the classification of the tumor, especially in cases of poorly differentiated carcinomas. Valuable information can also be obtained using ancillary intraoperative cytologic techniques, including fine needle aspirations, touch imprints, or scrapes, since cytologic preparations provide clear nuclear and cytoplasmic details without freezing artifact. The most problematic cases are borderline tumors and low-grade mucinous tumors; frozen section analysis of such tumors has a significantly lower sensitivity (33–87%) and specificity when compared to benign ovarian tumors and carcinomas. The most common underdiagnosed tumor type is borderline mucinous tumors, while the most common cause of overdiagnosis is misinterpretation of serous cystadenofibroma as borderline serous tumors. Surgical management of these neoplasms based on frozen section diagnosis should be used with caution. Studies demonstrate that the accuracy of frozen sections for the diagnosis of borderline tumors is lower than in frankly malignant tumors. However, frozen section

TABLE 6.6 Relative incidence of surface epithelial stromal tumors of ovary.

Serous neoplasms	46%
Mucinous neoplasms	36%
Endometrioid neoplasms	8%
Clear cell neoplasms	3%
Transitional neoplasms	2%
Undifferentiated neoplasms	2%
Mixed neoplasms	3%

Modified from Nucci MR, Oliva E. Gynecologic pathology. London: Elsevier Churchill Livingstone; 2009 (Volume in the series foundations in diagnostic pathology). Used with permission

TABLE 6.7 Relative incidence of surface epithelial carcinoma of ovary.

Serous cystadenocarcinoma	42%
Mucinous cystadenocarcinoma	12%
Endometrioid carcinoma	15%
Clear cell carcinoma	6%
Undifferentiated carcinoma	17%
Mixed	3%

Copeland LJ. Epithelial ovarian cancer. In: DiSaia PJ, Creasman WT, editors. Clinical gynecologic oncology. 7th ed. Philadelphia, PA: Mosby-Elsevier; 2007. Used with permission

evaluation identifying a borderline ovarian malignancy is accurate in excluding a benign condition which does not require further sampling for staging.

When the frozen section indicates the presence of a frankly invasive or malignant epithelial tumor, the optimal surgical procedure is hysterectomy with bilateral salpingooophorectomy. A complete abdominal exploration is performed, including an evaluation of all peritoneal intestinal surfaces, and any suspicious areas are biopsied. In patients with advanced lesions, including stage IIB, III, and stage IV, debulking or cytoreduction can be beneficial. Neoadjuvant chemotherapy is utilized in cases with advanced ovarian cancer where the likelihood of resectability is low. Cytomorphologic changes, such as bizarre nuclei and extensive tumor necrosis, should be considered at the time of intraoperative consultation of such cases, as will be discussed at the end of this chapter.

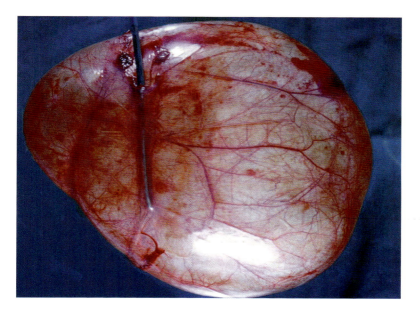

FIGURE 6.11 Serous cystadenoma: The outer surface of the unilocular cyst is smooth and lacks any excrescences. Blood vessels can be seen through the thin wall.

Serous Neoplasms

Most of these neoplasms are cystic or partially cystic. They contain clear serous fluid and have a variable amount of a fibrous tissue stromal component, hence the terms adenofibroma and cystadenofibroma. Serous cysts are lined by tall, columnar, ciliated, epithelial cells which form papillary structures with a vascular core. Psammoma bodies are often seen within the connective tissue cores or covered by the epithelial cells (Figs. 6.11–6.21, inclusive). Surface papillae may be seen on the surface of the ovary, but these can be benign and do not establish a diagnosis of borderline or frank malignancy. Differentiation between benign and frankly malignant serous tumors is not problematic in most cases. The main differential diagnosis is between benign and borderline tumors, since the latter warrant more extensive surgery or sampling.

Low-grade serous adenocarcinomas account for less than 10% of serous carcinomas. They commonly present with a component of serous borderline tumor. Differentiating high-grade serous

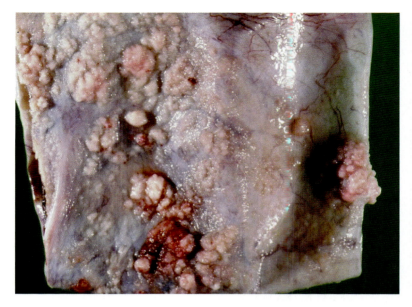

FIGURE 6.12 Serous cystadenoma: The inner surface shows a few papillae. The epithelial proliferation is not as lush as seen in borderline tumors.

carcinoma from other high-grade surface epithelial tumors such as endometrioid or clear cell carcinomas is not critical at the time of frozen section evaluation. It requires routine sampling and careful evaluation of multiple areas of the mass on permanent sections. Metastatic lesions should also be considered in the differential diagnosis of high-grade carcinomas; clinical history and immunohistochemical stains are often necessary to make this distinction. The key features of serous tumors are summarized below.

Key Features of Benign Serous Tumors (Figs. 6.11–6.14)
- Unilocular or multilocular cysts containing clear watery fluid
- Range in size from 1 to 10 cm (less than 1 cm is classified as inclusion cyst)
- Bilateral in 10–20% of cases
- Cyst wall is thin and often transparent
- Epithelial lining mostly ciliated with a few secretory cells
- Epithelium lacks significant cytologic nuclear atypia
- Papillae lack significant architectural atypia or complexity
- Variable amount of stromal component

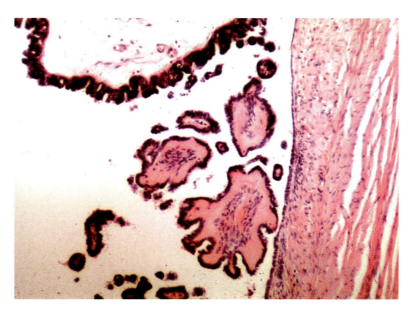

FIGURE 6.13 Serous cystadenoma: The papillae are covered by single layer of ciliated columnar epithelium, and a few psammoma bodies can be identified (H&E, medium power).

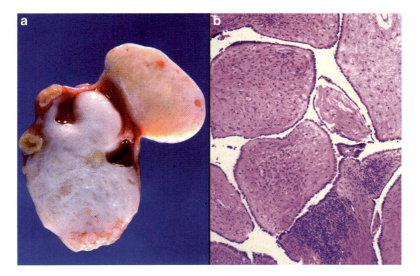

FIGURE 6.14 Serous cystadenofibroma: (**a**) Solid areas are not an indication of malignancy, but should be thoroughly sampled to exclude such a possibility (H&E, low power). (**b**) The stroma is a major component of the mass. Nuclear atypia is lacking in the epithelial and stromal cells (H&E, low power).

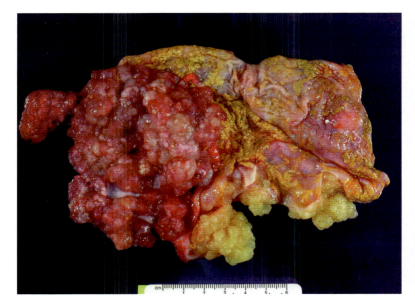

FIGURE 6.15 Serous borderline tumor: Lush papillary proliferations fill the cyst and are also seen on the surface. Thorough sampling of multiple areas to rule out foci of frankly invasive malignancy is critical. Borderline tumors are often bilateral.

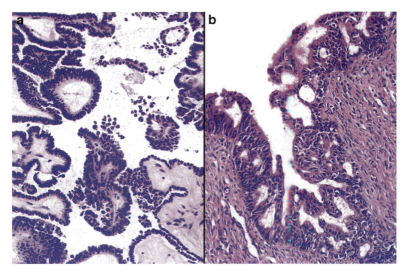

FIGURE 6.16 Serous borderline tumor: (**a**) and (**b**) Complex branching of the papillae and the stratification of the epithelial cells, usually limited to three layers, differentiates this from benign serous neoplasms. Cells may have cilia. Nuclear atypia is mild and mitotic figures are rare (H&E, medium power).

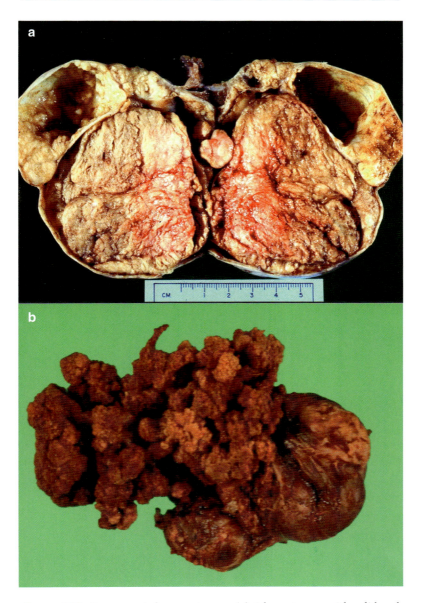

FIGURE 6.17 Serous cystadenocarcinoma: (**a**) A large tumor, with solid and cystic areas, foci of hemorrhage, and necrosis. The cyst has thick walls and septae. (**b**) Another tumor adjoining a benign cyst. Sections from the transition of the benign cyst and the solid components help in determining the serous nature of a poorly differentiated carcinoma.

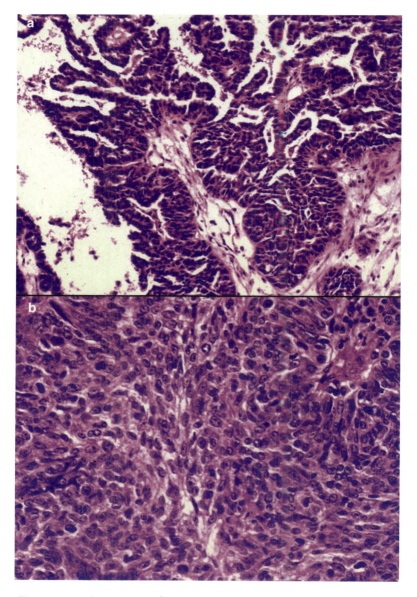

FIGURE 6.18 Serous cystadenocarcinoma: (**a**) Marked stratification of the epithelial cells covering complex papillae (H&E, medium power). (**b**) A poorly differentiated carcinoma with marked nuclear atypia and areas of solid growth pattern that invade the stroma (H&E, high power).

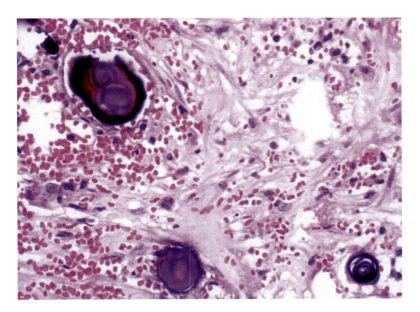

FIGURE 6.19 Serous carcinoma of the peritoneum: The peritoneum was studded with many nodules of variable size, showing papillary deposits of serous carcinoma, with psammoma bodies. Differentiation from metastatic ovarian serous tumors is not feasible on the frozen section, and it depends on the lack of involvement of ovaries, which were of normal size and showed no evidence of tumor (H&E, medium power).

Key Features of Serous Borderline Tumors (Figs. 6.15 and 6.16)
- Large cystic lesions, often bilateral (25–30%)
- Fluid content is usually serous but occasionally mucinous
- Surface papillary excrescences (50%)
- Numerous broad fronds and lush papillae filling some cysts
- Complex branching pattern of fine velvet like papillae, tufting, and "detached" budding
- Can have micropapillary foci with long thin papillae
- Cellular stratification up to three layers
- Nuclear atypia is mild to focally moderate at most
- Rare mitotic figure with altered distribution

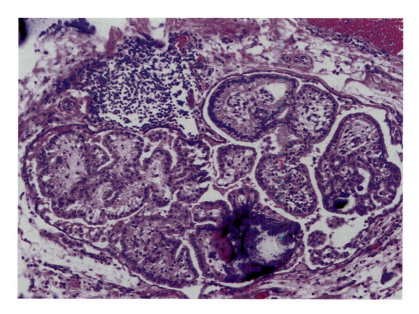

FIGURE 6.20 Noninvasive peritoneal implant: A well circumscribed nest of papillae with a psammoma body. The epithelial cells do not show nuclear atypia (H&E, medium power).

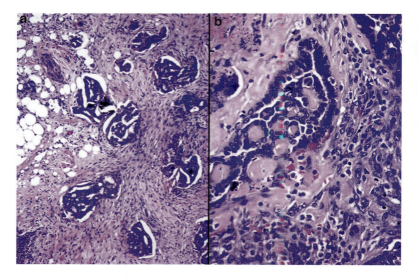

FIGURE 6.21 Invasive peritoneal implants: (a) and (b) Deep destructive invasion by irregular nests of epithelial cells with marked nuclear atypia. The nests have tentacular outline, in contrast to the smooth outline of noninvasive implants illustrated in the previous figure, and often induce a desmoplastic response in the stroma (H&E, medium power).

Key Features of Serous Adenocarcinoma (Figs. 6.17 and 6.18)
- Large, complex, solid, and cystic masses
- Bilateral in two thirds of cases
- Most patients present with extraovarian spread
- Cysts with irregular and thick septae
- Solid nodules with necrosis and/or hemorrhage
- Complex branching papillae, glands, or solid sheets of cells
- Marked stratification (>3 layers), marked nuclear atypia
- Destructive stromal invasion with desmoplasia and necrosis
- Capsular or vascular invasion

Serous Carcinoma of the Peritoneum

These neoplasms predominantly involve the peritoneal surface with minimal or no involvement of the ovaries. Differentiation between these tumors and ovarian serous tumors depends on the gross operative findings of the extent and location of the tumor. Frozen sections confirm the serous papillary nature of the deposits, but do not help to differentiate between these two neoplasms, since their histomorphologic and cytomorphologic features are similar (Fig. 6.19).

Key Features of Serous Carcinoma of the Peritoneum
- Rare, usually elderly women
- Diffuse involvement of peritoneum
- Superficial invasion of ovaries is absent or minimal
- Histology similar to ovarian serous carcinoma

Peritoneal Implants

Over 50% of patients with surface tumors have implants (Segal and Hart 1992). These are often sampled to determine if they are noninvasive (Fig. 6.20) or invasive (Fig. 6.21); the presence of the latter type has a negative impact on the prognosis. The key features of each type are listed below.

Key Features of Noninvasive Implants
- Well defined deposits with a few glands, papillae, and small epithelial nests
- Nests extend into fibrous septa between fat lobules, but maintain well defined contours
- Small submesothelial spaces filled with papillae
- Desmoplastic type shows fibrous nests plastered on surface and minimal epithelial component
- Lacks irregular destructive invasion of the underlying stroma
- Hierarchical branching of papillae
- Minimal nuclear atypia and only rare mitotic figure, if any
- Psammoma bodies frequent

Key Features of Invasive Implants
- Destructive invasion of deep omental or visceral adipose tissues by glands and small nests with irregular tentacular contours
- The nests incorporate adipose tissue and extend beyond the fibrous stroma
- Individual cells or clusters infiltrating stroma, often surrounded by artifactual stromal retraction or space with no lining
- Epithelial cells are dominant and disorderly distributed
- More significant nuclear atypia, similar to low-grade carcinoma, with mitotic figures
- Stromal desmoplasia

Mucinous Neoplasms

Mucinous carcinomas were considered to be the third most common type of ovarian carcinoma, comprising 6–25% of all primary surface epithelial tumors. However, the frequency of primary mucinous carcinomas of ovary is probably much lower than previously reported, encompassing <3% of ovarian carcinomas (Seidman 2003). The tumors are cystic or partially cystic, and usually multilocular (Fig. 6.22). They contain viscid mucinous material and are lined by tall, columnar, mucin-producing epithelium. In the majority of cases, the epithelium is of intestinal type, including goblet cells, some gastric and, occasionally, neuroendocrine or Paneth cells. A smaller number of cases has endocervical type of tall, columnar epithelium (Fig. 6.23). Although papillae may be encountered, they are less prominent than in the case of serous tumors. Similar to serous tumors, a variable amount of fibrous tissue component is present and such neoplasms are referred to as adenofibromas or cystadenofibromas (Fig. 6.24).

Key Features of Primary Benign Mucinous Tumors
- Large unilateral cystic mass
- Usually multilocular smooth lined bluish white cysts
- Cysts lined by intestinal type (goblet) or endocervical type (tall columnar mucinous) epithelium
- Lack of nuclear atypia
- May have a serous or Brenner component and, rarely, mature teratoma
- May coexist with borderline or malignant mucinous component

Differentiation of benign from borderline and frankly malignant mucinous tumors may present a problem at the time of surgical intraoperative consultation. The key features of these three categories are listed below. In some cases, it is not possible to distinguish benign

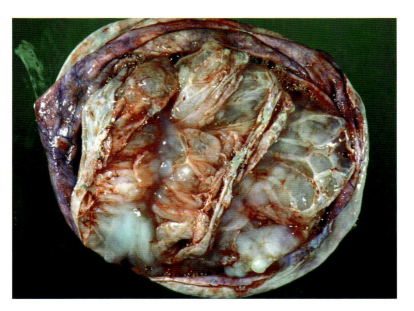

FIGURE 6.22 Mucinous cystadenoma: The cystic neoplasm is multiloculated and contains mucoid material. Tumor size is not an indication of malignancy, since some of the largest tumors we encountered were benign cystadenomas. From Ramzy I. Essentials of gynecologic and obstetric pathology. Norwalk: Appleton Century Crofts; 1983. p. 257. Used with permission.

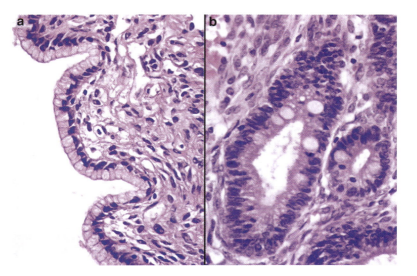

FIGURE 6.23 Mucinous cystadenoma: (**a**) A single layer of tall columnar endocervical type epithelium lines the cyst (H&E, medium power). (**b**) Intestinal type epithelium with goblet cells (H&E, medium power).

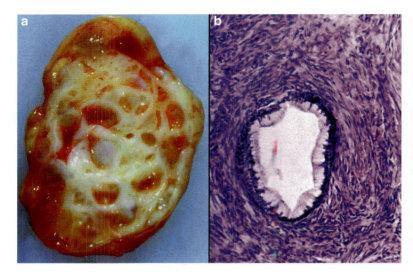

FIGURE 6.24 Mucinous cystadenofibroma: (**a**) Multiple cysts are seen within the fibrous background (H&E, low power). (**b**) The cysts are lined by goblet-type mucinous cells (H&E, low power).

mucinous tumors from borderline lesions at time of frozen sections, due to tangential sectioning or because of focal proliferative features. In this situation, it is advisable to defer diagnosis, rendering a preliminary diagnosis of "mucinous neoplasm; cannot rule out borderline tumor." When a borderline component is identified, but accounts for less than 10% of the tumor, the term "mucinous cystadenoma with focal proliferation" or focal atypia may be utilized.

Nuclear atypia is usually minimal or mild, even in borderline neoplasms. The presence of severe nuclear atypia merits the diagnosis of mucinous borderline tumor with intraepithelial (intraglandular) carcinoma. The possibility of metastatic carcinoma should also be considered in cases with significant nuclear atypia. Microinvasive carcinoma in borderline tumors can be identified as single cells or small nests infiltrating the stroma. However, recognition at the time of frozen section of intraepithelial carcinoma component and/or determination of microinvasion is not critical, since management of these neoplasms is identical to that of borderline tumors without these components. Furthermore, multiple sections are often required to identify such foci (Figs. 6.25 and 6.26).

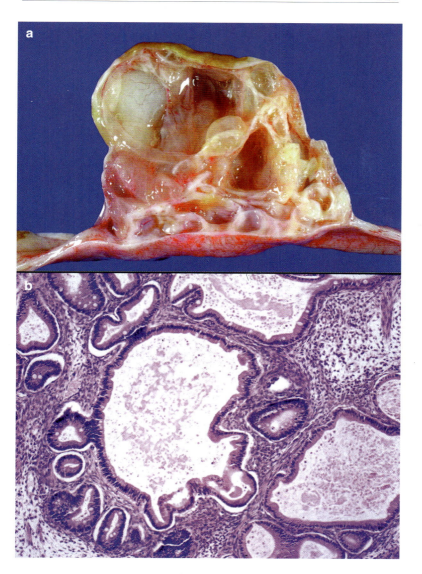

FIGURE 6.25 Mucinous tumor of borderline malignancy: (**a**) A solid area in the wall of a large multiloculated cyst (H&E, low power). (**b**) Small daughter cysts are budding from the large cyst (H&E, low power).

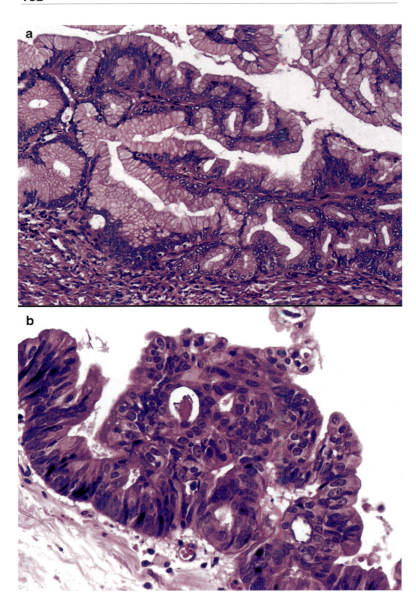

FIGURE 6.26 Mucinous tumor of borderline malignancy: (**a**) Papillae with complex architecture and stratification to two or three cell layers (H&E, low power). (**b**) Mild nuclear atypia and mitotic figures away from the basal layer are seen (H&E, medium power).

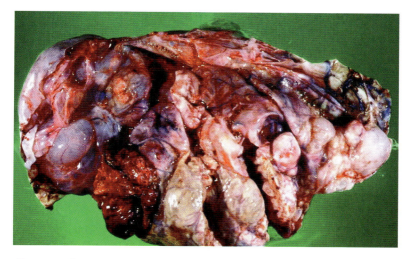

FIGURE 6.27 Mucinous cystadenocarcinoma: Large cystic tumor with irregularly thick septae and solid areas. Note areas of hemorrhage and necrosis. The malignant change may be focal, and adequate sampling is necessary. From Ramzy I. Essentials of gynecologic and obstetric pathology. Norwalk: Appleton Century Crofts; 1983. p. 259. Used with permission.

Frankly invasive mucinous carcinomas have complex gland architecture, significant cytologic atypia and larger areas of stromal invasion (>5 mm in linear extent or 10 mm^2 in area). Stromal invasion in primary mucinous carcinomas is characterized most commonly by an expansile growth pattern rather than an infiltrative growth pattern (Figs. 6.27 and 6.28).

Intestinal type mucinous adenocarcinomas should be differentiated from metastatic carcinomas of gastrointestinal origin and the features that help in clarifying this are also listed below.

Key Features of Mucinous Borderline Tumors
- Large unilateral cystic mass
- Multilocular cysts with finer honey-comb pattern
- Large cysts are surrounded by small "daughter" cysts
- Papillary folds demonstrating variable complexity of architecture
- Stratification of epithelial lining into 2–3 layers
- Mild cytologic atypia
- Altered distribution of mitotic figures, some away from the basal layers

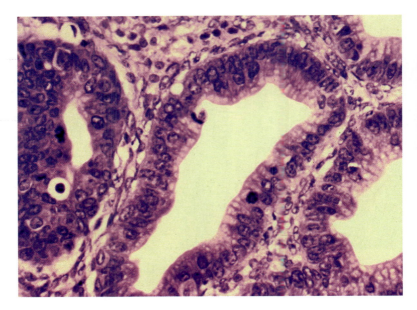

FIGURE 6.28 Mucinous adenocarcinoma: Irregular glands, arranged haphazardly and inducing desmoplastic stromal reaction. Papillary formations are more prominent in endocervical type than the intestinal type. Nuclear atypia is evident and mitotic figures are easily identified (H&E, medium power). From Ramzy I. Essentials of gynecologic and obstetric pathology. Norwalk: Appleton Century Crofts; 1983. p. 260. Used with permission.

Key Features of Primary Mucinous Adenocarcinoma
- Large (>10 cm) complex unilateral solid and cystic mass
- Irregular thick cyst wall with septations and solid nodules with necrosis
- Often demonstrate coexistence of benign, borderline, and invasive carcinoma components
- Complex architecture with cribriform or irregular glands
- Expansile invasion or less commonly destructive stromal invasion with necrosis and desmoplasia
- Marked cytologic atypia and frequent mitosis
- Intestinal type tends to have fewer papillae than endocervical type
- Endocervical type often associated with serous elements and pelvic endometriosis

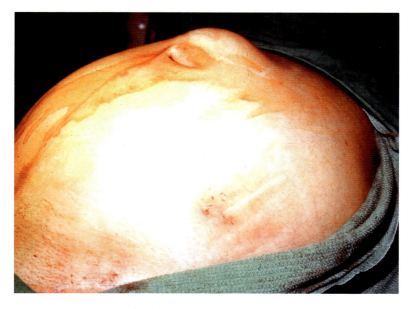

FIGURE 6.29 Peritoneal adenomucinosis: The abdomen is distended with mucinous material. This patient had recurrent episodes every 3–4 years. Slide courtesy of Dr. Hugh H. Allen, London, Canada.

Peritoneal Adenomucinosis (Pseudomyxoma Peritoneii)

These are benign or borderline neoplastic mucinous glands and free mucin that dissect between fibrous and omental tissues. They are only seen in association with benign and malignant mucinous tumors of intestinal type, particularly borderline lesions (15%) and are not an indicator of ovarian cancer. The majority of recurrent cases are associated with mucinous tumors of appendix (Figs. 6.29 and 6.30).

Endometrioid Tumors

These are only responsible for less than 10% of the primary surface epithelial neoplasms of the ovary. Most of the cases are malignant, with fewer cases of borderline and benign tumors in the form of cystadenoma, adenofibroma, or cystadenofibroma (Figs. 6.31–6.33). Endometrioid borderline tumors are responsible for about 20% of endometrioid tumors of the ovary, and a third of cases are associated with uterine endometrial hyperplasia or a second primary carcinoma of the uterine body. Focal microinvasion does not appear to affect the prognosis.

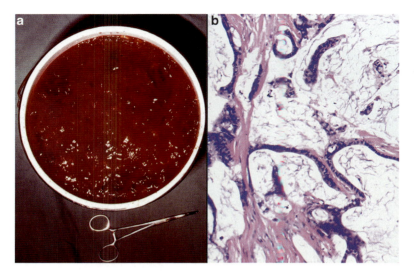

FIGURE 6.30 Peritoneal adenomucinosis: (**a**) Abundant mucoid gelatinous material removed from the abdominal cavity of the patient depicted in the previous figure (H&E, low power). (**b**) Pools of mucin are sparsely cellular, with a few glands. Examination of the appendix is critical, since many cases are associated with mucinous lesions of the appendix (H&E, low power).

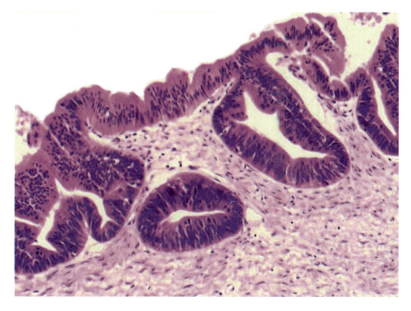

FIGURE 6.31 Endometrioid adenofibroma: A fibrous stroma separates glands of endometrial type (H&E, medium power).

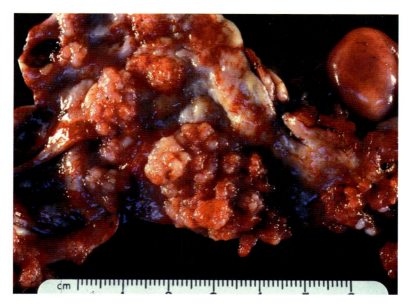

FIGURE 6.32 Endometrioid tumor: The cyst has lush papillae and solid areas. Frank malignancy was suspected on the basis of the gross appearance. Extensive sampling, however, failed to demonstrate evidence of any invasive component.

The great majority of endometrioid surface epithelial tumors are well to moderately differentiated carcinomas (grades 1 and 2). Differential diagnosis of endometrioid adenocarcinoma to be considered at the time of frozen section is with other ovarian tumors, such as sex cord stromal tumors, carcinoid tumors, and with metastatic colon carcinoma. The presence of more typical endometrioid features such as squamous differentiation and intraluminal mucin supports an endometrioid carcinoma; the absence of salt and pepper chromatin or dirty necrosis differentiates endometrioid tumors from carcinoid and colonic neoplasms, respectively. Distinguishing high-grade endometrioid adenocarcinomas from serous adenocarcinomas is not critical at the time of frozen section, and the diagnosis of high-grade surface epithelial tumor can be rendered, deferring further classification, after additional permanent sections become available.

Key Features of Benign Endometrioid Tumors
- Unilateral, solid mass with small cysts
- Well spaced glands resembling endometrial type glands
- Background of fibrous stroma

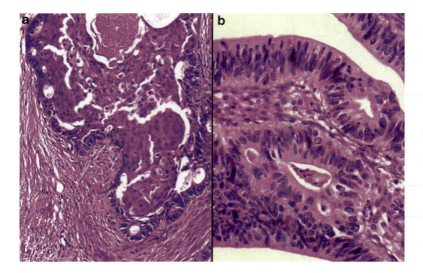

FIGURE 6.33 Endometrioid adenocarcinoma: (**a**) Irregular glands and solid nests, with focal squamous metaplasia infiltrate a desmoplastic stroma (H&E, medium power). (**b**) The cells are of endometrioid type, with nuclear atypia and stratification. Villoglandular pattern and presence of focal squamous metaplasia supports endometrioid differentiation (H&E, medium power).

Key Features of Borderline Endometrioid Tumors
- Unilateral or bilateral lesions
- Solid or partially cystic
- Atypical or histologically malignant endometrioid glands within a fibrous stroma or with a papillary architecture
- Lack stromal invasion

Key Features of Endometrioid Adenocarcinomas
- Cystic or solid with hemorrhage and necrosis
- Often demonstrate transition from benign, borderline to carcinoma
- Complex glandular, villoglandular, cribriform, or solid architecture
- Squamous, mucinous, ciliated, or secretory metaplasia can be present
- Destructive stromal invasion

Clear Cell Neoplasms

Most clear cell surface tumors are carcinomas (Fig. 6.34). Differential diagnosis includes other primary ovarian or metastatic tumors with clear or eosinophilic cells such as yolk sac tumor, endometrioid

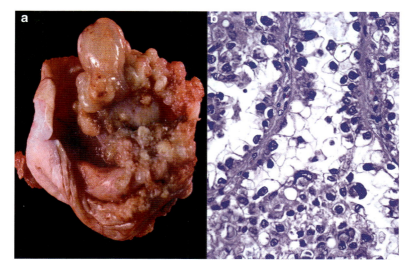

FIGURE 6.34 Clear cell carcinoma: (**a**) Cystic tumor, with thick walls and irregular papillary growth within the cyst. Necrosis and hemorrhage are often seen (H&E, medium power). (**b**) Cells with well defined borders and clear cytoplasm lining clefts and glandular spaces. The nuclei are pleomorphic with some hobnail pattern (H&E, medium power).

tumor with secretory change, juvenile granulosa cell tumor, or metastatic renal cell carcinoma. The key features of clear cell ovarian neoplasms are listed below.

Key Features of Benign and Borderline Clear Cell Tumors
- Unilateral, solid with small cysts
- Glands and tubules lined by flat, cuboidal cells, or hobnail cells with clear or eosinophilic cytoplasm
- Minimal or moderate atypia and rare mitosis
- Background fibrous stroma (adenofibroma)

Key Features of Clear Cell Carcinoma
- Unilateral cystic mass with thick walls
- Solid nodules with necrosis and hemorrhage
- Admixture of growth patterns: tubulocystic, papillary or solid architecture
- Polyhedral, cuboidal, or hobnail cells with clear to eosinophilic cytoplasm,
- Marked nuclear atypia, hyperchromasia, and mitotic activity

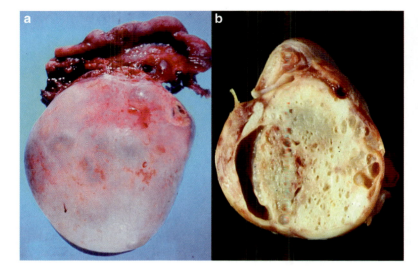

FIGURE 6.35 Transitional cell (Brenner) tumor: (**a**) A well defined firm solid tumor with a smooth outer surface (H&E, low power). (**b**) Occasional small cysts and mucinous cystadenoma may be associated with some transitional cell tumors (H&E, medium power). See also Fig. 6.9b.

Transitional Cell (Brenner) Tumors

This group encompasses benign, borderline, and malignant Brenner tumors, as well as non-Brenner transitional carcinoma. Brenner tumors are usually benign, well defined, fibroma-like solid nodules. They are often an incidental finding and rarely submitted for intraoperative consultation, unless there is a clinical reason for suspicion. The tumor is characterized by islands of uniform epithelial cells with nuclear "coffee-bean" folds, embedded in fibrous tissue. Small cysts lined by mucinous cells may be seen, and there is tendency to be associated with teratomas or mucinous neoplasms. Borderline (proliferating) Brenner tumors are large solid or partially cystic neoplasms, with stratification and nuclear pleomorphism of the epithelium lining the cysts and the papillae. Frankly malignant Brenner tumors are rare. They show necrosis, hemorrhage, prominent nuclear atypia, and an invasive growth pattern (Figs. 6.35–6.37).

Other Surface Epithelial Neoplasms

The surface epithelium of the ovary may develop malignancy in the form of mixed müllerian tumors. These consist of several mesenchymal and epithelial elements similar to those previously described

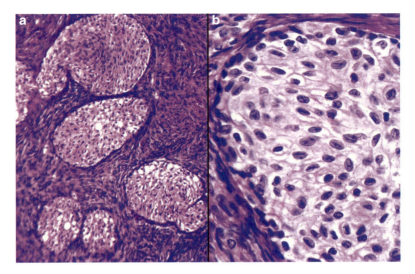

FIGURE 6.36 Transitional cell tumor: (**a**) Nests of transitional cells surrounded by fibrous stroma (H&E, low power). (**b**) The nuclei are uniform and show longitudinal "coffee-bean like" grooves (H&E, medium power).

under uterine corpus (Fig. 6.38). Such tumors behave aggressively and are usually encountered in postmenopausal women.

SEX CORD AND STROMAL TUMORS

Sex cord and stromal tumors account for approximately 5–10% of all ovarian neoplasms. The majority are either benign or of low potential for aggressive behavior and metastasis, and have favorable long term prognosis. Some of these tumors are hormonally active, accounting for 90% of all functional ovarian neoplasms. Most tumors are unilateral lesions, confined to the ovary, and in younger patients with stage Ia disease, unilateral salpingooophorectomy is the recommended procedure. Advanced stage disease, particularly in older patients, is managed with complete staging and hysterectomy with bilateral salpingooophorectomy. Estrogen producing tumors are associated with endometrial hyperplasia or carcinoma; thus, surgical evaluation should include dilatation and curettage of the uterine cavity.

The neoplasms are usually solid or partially cystic, and in steroid secreting tumors, there is a characteristic brown, orange or

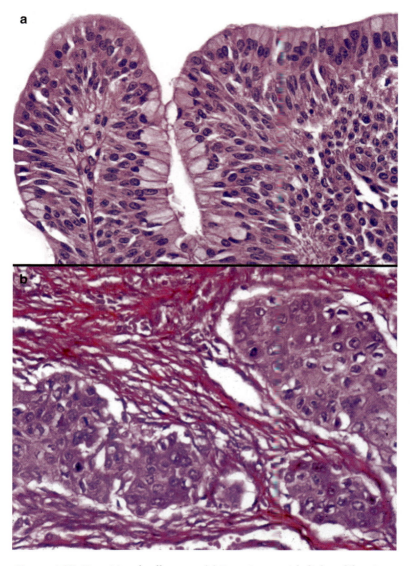

FIGURE 6.37 Transitional cell tumor: (**a**) Prominent epithelial proliferation, papillae and focal mucinous differentiation are not uncommon in borderline (proliferating) tumors (H&E, medium power). (**b**) Malignant transitional cell tumor with nuclear pleomorphism, an infiltrative pattern and areas of necrosis (H&E, medium power).

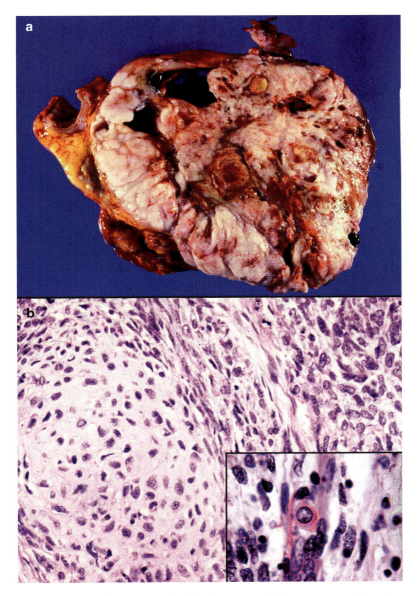

FIGURE 6.38 Malignant mixed müllerian tumor: (**a**) Large tumor with variegated colors and consistency, showing necrosis and hemorrhage. (**b**) A mixture of malignant epithelial and stromal tissues, including cartilage is evident. Some striated muscle is illustrated in *inset* (H&E, high power, oil).

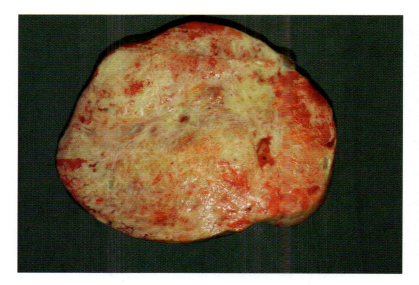

FIGURE 6.39 Theca cell tumor: Sex cord/stromal neoplasms tend to be solid tumors with a *yellow*, *orange* or *brown* color, reflecting steroid hormone content. Although a combination of granulosa and theca cells is fairly common, this tumor showed only theca cells without any granulosa cell component.

yellow color, reflecting its lipid-rich content (Figs. 6.39 and 6.40). Staining of a frozen section with oil red O often demonstrates the presence of small intracytoplasmic lipid droplets, as illustrated later under the discussion of Theca cell neoplasms. Sex cord and stromal neoplasms may show evidence of differentiation into granulosa, theca, Sertoli, or interstitial Leydig cell lines. Tumors showing dual components such as granulosa and theca cell, or Sertoli–Leydig cell elements, are often encountered. Gynandroblastoma is a rare tumor where granulosa and Sertoli–Leydig elements are present. Definitive classification of these rare types requires multiple sampling on permanent sections.

Granulosa Cell Tumors

These are the most commonly encountered sex cord neoplasms in women, accounting for 2% of ovarian tumors. Over half the patients are postmenopausal, with a peak age of 45–55 years. The clinical presentation depends on the hormonal activity of the neoplasm and the age of the patient, and is usually in the form of abnormal

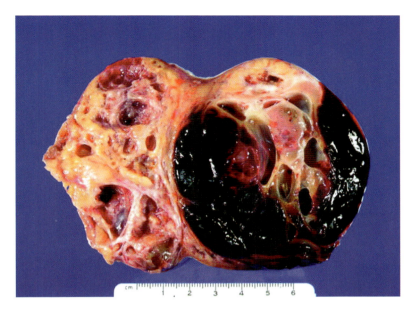

FIGURE 6.40 Granulosa cell tumor: The partially cystic tumor shows areas of hemorrhage and *orange* hue.

vaginal bleeding as a result of hyperestronism, with some patients presenting with ascites or hemoperitoneum. In less than 5 % of cases, it is associated with an endometrioid adenocarcinoma of the uterine body and 25–50% of cases are associated with endometrial hyperplasia. A wide variety of admixed histologic patterns are encountered, including solid, sarcomatoid, trabecular, insular, follicular, watered silk (moiré), and gyriform (Figs. 6.41 and 6.42). In the microfollicular pattern, rosette structures reminiscent of Call Exner bodies can be encountered, facilitating the diagnosis. Intraoperative cytologic preparations are beneficial, demonstrating the characteristic granulosa cells with scant cytoplasm, uniform and angular to oval, often grooved "coffee bean-like" nuclei (Fig. 6.43). The stroma may be luteinized. Tumors occurring in children and juveniles may be associated with Maffucci and other syndromes. They tend to be hemorrhagic, with the formation of large cystic areas (Fig. 6.44). Although the juvenile granulosa cells can demonstrate frequent mitotic figures, they behave less aggressively than the adult type.

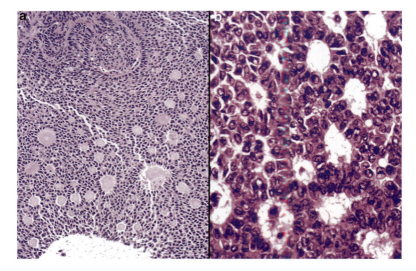

FIGURE 6.41 Granulosa cell tumor: (**a**) Neoplastic cells form rosettes and small cysts. Identification of areas with Call Exner like rosettes is quite helpful in supporting the diagnosis (H&E, low power). (**b**) Granulosa cells have scant cytoplasm, uniform round to oval nuclei, some with nuclear grooves. The rosettes are not true acini; their center contains degenerated cells with nuclear and cytoplasmic debris (H&E, medium power).

Key Features of Adult Granulosa Cell Tumors
- Unilateral, solid or solid/cystic lesions
- Yellow white cut surface with areas of hemorrhage
- Solid, trabecular, microfollicular, insular, watered silk and gyriform patterns
- Fibrothecomatous background which may be luteinized
- Cells with scant cytoplasm, round to oval nuclei with grooves
- Minimal cytologic atypia and low mitotic rate

Key Features of Juvenile Granulosa Cell Tumors
- Unilateral, solid, and cystic mass
- Lobulated gray white to tan yellow surface with occasional hemorrhage and necrosis
- Diffuse or nodular architecture
- Moderate to abundant eosinophilic to clear cytoplasm and hyperchromatic nuclei lacking nuclear grooves
- Can demonstrate marked nuclear atypia and brisk mitotic activity

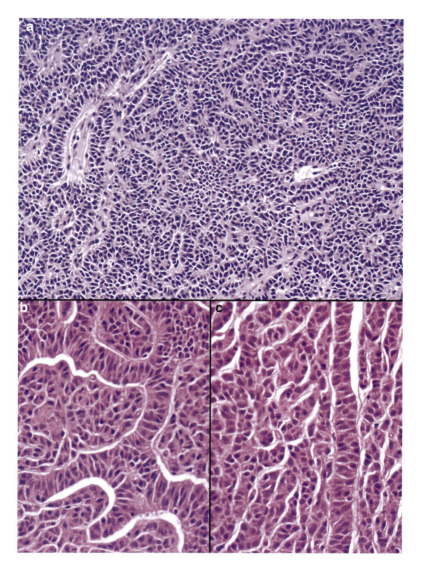

FIGURE 6.42 Granulosa cell tumor: (**a–c**) The trabecular pattern dominates this peritoneal nodule, resected from the surface of the small intestine 20 years after salpingooophorectomy for a granulosa cell tumor of the right ovary. The neoplastic cells are fairly uniform, without evidence of active mitosis. The cells may form thin trabeculae, resulting in a "watered silk" appearance [(**a**): H&E, low power; (**b**) and (**c**): H&E, medium power].

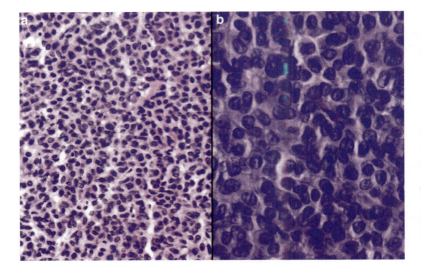

Figure 6.43 Granulosa cell tumor: (a) Neoplastic cells arranged diffusely in a sarcomatoid or solid pattern. Note the difficulty in identifying classic rosettes in this frozen section (H&E, medium power). (b) The cells have scant cytoplasm and some nuclear grooves, although grooves may be difficult to appreciate in thick sections (H&E, high power).

Most granulosa cell tumors are low-grade malignancies, with only 5% of stage I cases recurring. Recurrences often appear more than 5 years after the initial therapy. Adverse prognostic factors include large tumor size (>5 cm), bilateral involvement, intraabdominal rupture, nuclear atypia, and high mitotic rate. However, the single most important prognostic factor is stage, and the presence of residual disease. Any temptation to predict the behavior of granulosa cell tumors on the basis of frozen sections should be strongly resisted, since such behavior cannot be linked to specific histologic parameters, even after additional sampling for permanent sections. Differential diagnoses to consider at the time of frozen section are other primary ovarian or metastatic carcinomas, transitional cell carcinoma or undifferentiated carcinomas. Ovarian carcinoids show "salt and pepper" chromatin pattern and lack nuclear grooves, their cytoplasm is immunoreactive to neuroendocrine markers, and other teratomatous elements may be present. Endometrioid adenocarcinoma lacks the Call Exner bodies, nuclear grooves, and may show squamous metaplasia. Transitional cell carcinomas typically

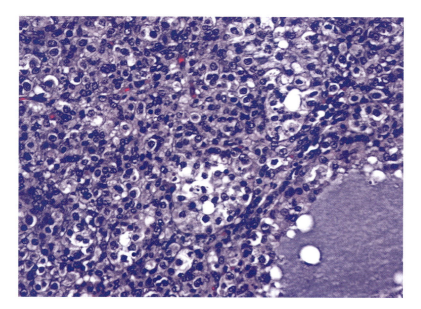

FIGURE 6.44 Juvenile granulosa cell tumor: The cells are diffusely arranged, and have moderate to abundant amounts of cytoplasm. Cystic areas are often seen and focal luteinization of the neoplastic cells can be seen. The nuclei show atypia and lack nuclear grooves. Despite brisk mitotic activity, juvenile granulosa cell tumors behave less aggressively than the adult type (H&E, medium power).

have high-grade nuclei, mitosis, and extensive necrosis. Poorly differentiated carcinomas and sarcomas show evidence of active mitosis that is lacking in adult granulosa cell tumors. Markers for melanoma differentiate its amelanotic variant from granulosa cell tumors. Small cell carcinoma with hypercalcemia, unlike juvenile granulosa cell tumors, shows necrosis and is not immunoreactive to inhibin. Yolk sac tumor can also be considered in the differential diagnosis of juvenile granulose cell tumor. However, yolk sac tumors are typically characterized by a more primitive appearance of the nuclei and a very loose stromal background.

Theca Cell Tumor and Fibroma

This group of ovarian neoplasms represents the most commonly encountered sex stromal tumors, accounting for approximately 4% of all ovarian tumors. It encompasses typical, luteinized, and malignant theca cell tumors, fibroma and fibrosarcoma, as well as

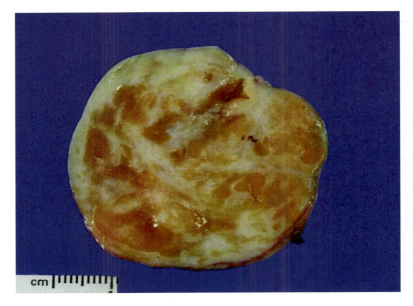

FIGURE 6.45 Fibrothecoma: Most neoplasms of the fibrothecoma group are solid firm masses, with a smooth outer surface and a *yellowish white* cut surface, depending on the fibrous and lipid content of the tumor.

sclerosing stromal tumor. Typical thecomas occur in postmenopausal women, and are often associated with estrogenic changes. Up to 37% are associated with endometrial hyperplasia and 25% of postmenopausal patients with thecomas have an associated endometrial adenocarcinoma or, rarely, a malignant mixed müllerian tumor, or endometrial stromal sarcoma. Highly luteinized tumors have a tendency to be androgenic. Theca cell tumors tend to be unilateral, solid with an orange or yellow cut surface, and occasionally may be cystic. The spindled neoplastic cells have abundant lipid-rich cytoplasm and staining of a frozen section demonstrates oil red O positive material within the cytoplasmic vacuoles (Figs. 6.45 and 6.46). The luteinized stromal cells can form nests within an edematous background. Theca cell tumors are immunoreactive to inhibin and vimentin, unlike fibromas which react only to vimentin. Differentiating fibromas from thecomas, however, is of little practical value at the time of frozen section, and rendering a diagnosis of fibrothecoma is appropriate. A combination of theca cells and granulosa cell elements is not uncommon (Fig. 6.47).

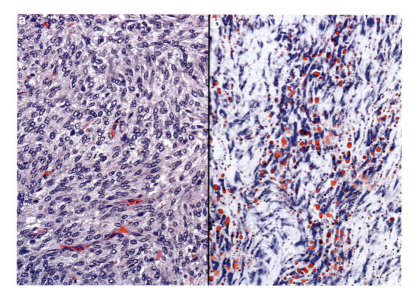

FIGURE 6.46 Theca cell tumor: (**a**) Plump spindled cells arranged in a wavy fascicular pattern or as nests. They have a lipid rich pale or vacuolated clear cytoplasm. (**b**) Oil red O staining of a frozen section is helpful in confirming the presence of intracellular lipid in sex cord/stromal neoplasms (Oil-red O, medium power).

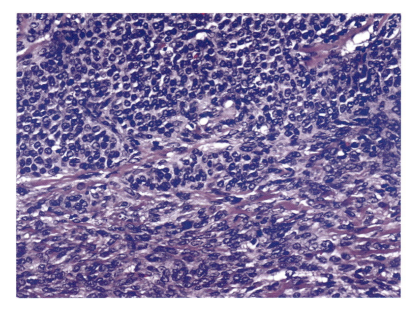

FIGURE 6.47 Granulosa Theca cell tumor: There is a mixture of granulosa and theca cell components in this tumor (H&E, medium power).

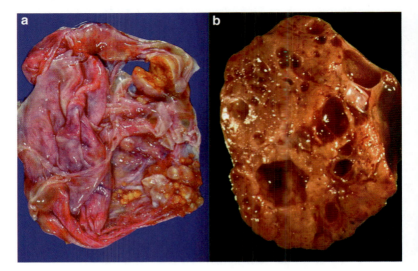

FIGURE 6.48 Sertoli and Leydig cell tumors: (**a**) Cystic neoplasm in a postmenopausal patient with evidence of virilization. Most of these tumors, however, are predominantly solid. (**b**) A tumor resected from a 5 year old girl presenting with 3 months history of precocious puberty and vaginal bleeding. Note the *brown-yellow* color and the presence of cystic areas in the predominantly solid neoplasm (Figs. 6.48b and 6.50 are from Ramzy I, Bos C. Sertoli cell tumors of ovary; light microscopic and ultrastructural study with histogenetic considerations. Cancer. 1976;38:2447–56, by permission).

Key Features of Theca Cell Tumors
- Postmenopausal women, may be virilizing
- Unilateral solid, orange, or yellow mass
- Plump spindled cells arranged in wavy bundles or nests
- Cytoplasm with vacuoles containing lipid
- Immunoreactive to inhibin
- Association with endometrial hyperplasia or carcinoma

Almost all pure thecomas are benign. Large lesions, however, require extensive sampling to rule out a fibrous component with malignant transformation. Such a change is usually in the form of fibrosarcoma, characterized by increased cellularity, nuclear atypia, mitotic activity, hemorrhage, or necrosis. Metastasis is rare, even in the presence of nuclear atypia and frequent mitosis.

Sclerosing stromal tumors: This is a benign tumor affecting young women (20–40 years). It is characterized by sclerosing nodules with some scattered clear cells. It is often associated with

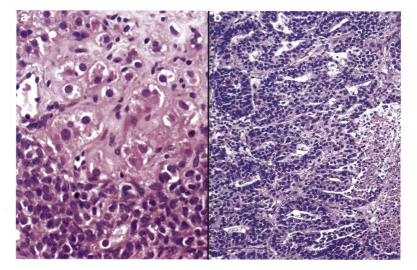

FIGURE 6.49 Sertoli–Leydig cell tumor: (**a**) The stroma contains nests of polygonal to round Leydig cells with abundant clear or pale cytoplasm. Sertoli cells have scant cytoplasm and dark nuclei with dense chromatin and do not show tubule formation in this section. The 70 year old patient showed signs of virilization. The presence of Sertoli cell component helps differentiate these tumors from steroid cell and pure Leydig cell tumors, illustrated in Fig. 6.51. (**b**) Poorly differentiated neoplasm, showing some tubules, areas of diffuse pattern and foci of necrosis.

menstrual abnormalities due to estrogenic or androgenic stimulation. Unlike theca cell tumors, sclerosing stromal tumors show immunoreactivity to SMA.

Sertoli–Leydig Cell Tumor (Androblastoma)

Tumors of Sertoli–Leydig cell differentiation are uncommon, accounting for less than 0.2% of all ovarian tumors. They are typically unilateral solid or partially cystic lesions that are gray to yellow on the cut section (Fig. 6.48). They are usually confined to the ovary and most can be managed with unilateral salpingooophorectomy. These tumors often occur in younger women (mean age 25 years), and about a third of the patients present with virilization. Sertoli–Leydig cell tumors are classified according to the degree of differentiation and the presence of heterologous elements. Well differentiated Sertoli–Leydig cell tumors are characterized by a predominantly tubular pattern (Fig. 6.49). The empty tubules are lined by tall columnar Sertoli cells with basal nuclei, and are separated by fibrous bands. Leydig cells with eosinophilic cytoplasm and round nuclei are seen within the stroma; they are polyclonal and probably reactive. Moderate or poorly differentiated tumors often exhibit a variety of patterns, including solid cords or diffuse spindle sarcoma-like pattern. Slit-like structures, tubular spaces with intracystic polypoid projections (rete-like), may be dominant in some tumors. Similar to granulosa cell tumors, histomorphology does not correlate with the behavior of Sertoli–Leydig neoplasms, but stage II tumors, particularly the poorly differentiated ones, tend to behave aggressively.

Key Features of Sertoli–Leydig Tumors
- Unilateral, usually solid tan to orange bosselated mass
- Tubules or cysts lined by columnar cells with uniform elongated basal nuclei
- Nests of Leydig cells with clear or amphophilic lipid rich cytoplasm
- Diffuse spindle stroma cells, trabeculae, and solid cords in poorly differentiated tumors

Sertoli–Leydig cell tumors should be differentiated from steroid cell tumors and hilus cell tumors which may be also associated with virilization, as discussed below.

Other Sex Cord Stromal Neoplasms

Pure Sertoli cell, Leydig cell and steroid cell neoplasms are rare. Sampling of several areas is necessary to assure the absence of other components in such neoplasms. A detailed discussion of these tumors is beyond the scope of this text, since definitive classification should await thorough sampling through routine fixation and processing, but a review of some of the features is appropriate.

Sertoli cell tumor (Pure): This solid, smooth or lobulated neoplasm has a yellow to tan cut surface. Most tumors are estrogenic, some are androgenic, and a few secrete renin. Histologically, they are similar to Sertoli–Leydig cell neoplasms, except for the absence of any significant number of Leydig cells (Fig. 6.50). Immunostaining may be necessary to differentiate the poorly differentiated tumors from other spindle cell neoplasms. Most Sertoli cell tumors behave in a benign fashion, but those with cytologic atypia and increased mitotic activity can be aggressive.

Steroid cell tumor: This tumor is usually androgenic (50%), but may secrete estrogen, cortisol, and progesterone, or result in hypercalcemia. The tumors are usually large, solid or partially cystic, and

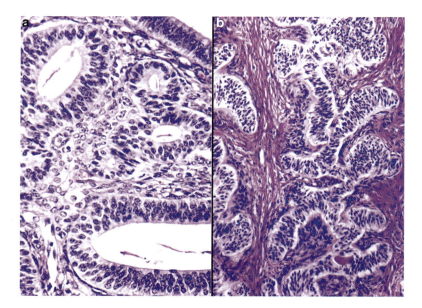

FIGURE 6.50 Sertoli cell tumor: (**a**) Well differentiated neoplasm, with cords and tubules lined by tall columnar cells. The elongated uniform nuclei are basally located and have small nucleoli. The fibrous stroma lacks Leydig cells (H&E, medium power). From Ramzy I. Essentials of gynecologic and obstetric pathology. Norwalk: Appleton Century Crofts; 1983. p. 286. Used with permission. (**b**) Trabeculae of sex cord cells arranged in a step-ladder fashion (H&E, low power).

occasionally show necrosis and hemorrhage. They are yellow/brown or black due to their lipid and lipochrome content respectively. Differential diagnosis includes Leydig cell tumor, hilus cell tumor, and stromal luteoma.

Leydig cell tumor: This rare tumor consists almost entirely of Leydig cells. It affects postmenopausal patients, and is usually androgenic, or associated with adrenal hyperplasia. The neoplastic cells possess bland nuclei and an eosinophilic or a lipid rich clear cytoplasm that may have Reinke crystals (Fig. 6.51). Nuclear atypia has no impact on behavior.

Hilus cell tumor: This is a neoplasm of Leydig like cells that is limited to the ovarian hilus. It may be associated with hyperplasia of the adjacent hilus cells and nerves.

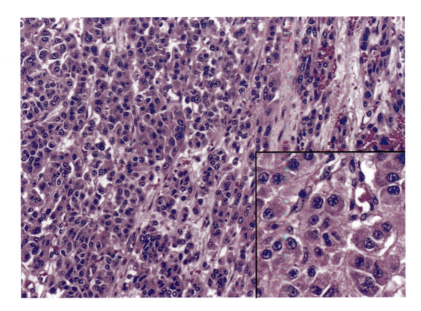

FIGURE 6.51 Leydig cell tumor. (a) and (b) The neoplastic cells have moderately to abundant eosinophilic cytoplasm, and central nuclei. Search for the characteristic Reinke crystalloid requires time and is not practical at the time of frozen section consultation (H&E, medium power; inset at higher magnification).

Benign signet ring stromal tumor: This rare solid tumor is characterized by signet ring cells that have bland nuclei pushed to the periphery by one or multiple vacuoles (Fig. 6.52). The neoplastic cells fail to form any acini, unlike those seen in Krukenberg tumors, and the vacuoles stain negatively for mucin or periodic acid Schiff. The cells are not reactive to keratin or CEA. The tumor is hormonally inert and no metastases have been reported.

Sex cord tumor with annular tubules (SCTAT): The histologic pattern of columnar cells arranged in annular tubular fashion around central hyaline material is fairly characteristic of this tumor, which is usually large and unilateral. It affects patients in their thirties (mean age 34 years) and behaves aggressively in 20% of cases. Patients with Peutz–Jeghers syndrome frequently have multiple small calcified tumorlets with similar histologic pattern in both ovaries, probably representing hamartomatous lesions, and these have a benign course (Fig. 6.53).

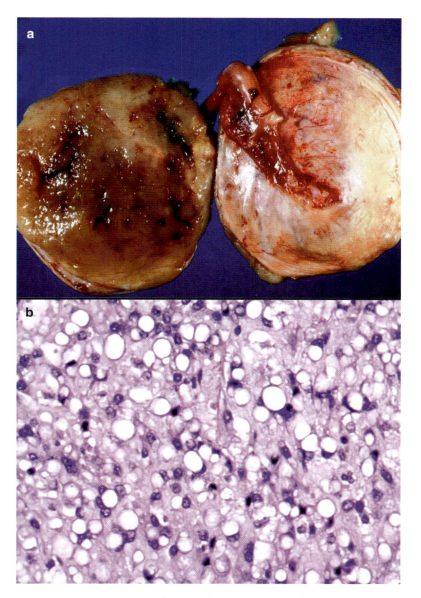

FIGURE 6.52 Signet-ring cell stromal tumor: (**a**) A solid neoplasm with smooth bosselated outer surface. (**b**) The signet ring cells have uniform bland nuclei, and the vacuoles lack lipid or glycogen, unlike those of Krukenberg tumors, illustrated in Fig. 6.70 (H&E, medium power) (From Ramzy I. Signet-ring stromal tumor of ovary: histochemical, light and electron microscopic study. Cancer. 1976;38:166–72, by permission).

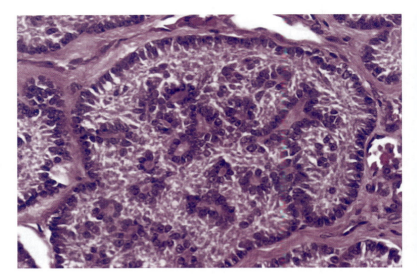

FIGURE 6.53 Sex cord tumor with annular tubules: The neoplastic cells form tubules around a central core of hyaline material (H&E, medium power).

GERM CELL NEOPLASMS

Neoplasms in this group show varying degrees of differentiation into embryonic and extra-embryonic tissues. They encompass dysgerminoma, teratomas (mature cystic and solid, immature and monodermal), embryonal carcinoma, yolk sac tumor, and nongestational choriocarcinoma. The tumors tend to occur in young patients, often below 40 years of age. They are responsible for 30–40% of primary ovarian tumors; 95% of these are mature cystic teratomas.

Mature Cystic Teratoma

This is the most common type of ovarian teratomas, representing 95% of germ cell neoplasms (dermoid cyst). They are often asymptomatic, discovered incidentally at laparotomy or during imaging, and rarely induce torsion or rupture, resulting in peritonitis. Mature cystic teratomas are bilateral in 15% of cases. The cyst contains semi-liquid sebaceous material, that solidifies at room temperature, and hair. At the time of intraoperative consultation, the cyst contents should be removed and the cyst wall inspected for architectural complexity or solid nodules "Rokitansky protuberance" (Figs. 6.54 and 6.55). Sections from the solid areas are most helpful in identifying the wide variety of mature tissues present that

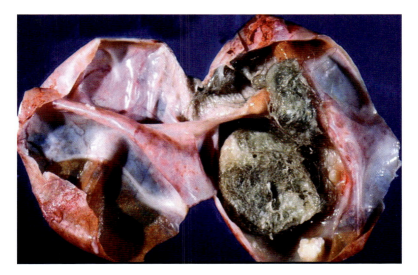

FIGURE 6.54 Mature cystic teratoma: The cystic neoplasm contains sebaceous material and hair. Sampling Rokitansky nodule helps to identify the variety of mature tissues derived from the three germ cell layers. From Ramzy I. Essentials of gynecologic and obstetric pathology. Norwalk: Appleton Century Crofts; 1983. p. 272. Used with permission.

are derived from the three germ cell layers, particularly ectodermal tissues. Occasionally, one tissue type forms the bulk of the teratoma, reflecting a monodermal differentiation. Examples include thyroid tissue in cases of struma ovarii and carcinoid differentiation, discussed below. Malignant transformation of mature cystic teratomas is rare (2%). It tends to occur in patients older than 40 years, resulting in large solid or fungating masses with necrosis and hemorrhage. These tumors are often squamous cell carcinomas, but other malignancies such as adenocarcinoma, neuroectodermal carcinoma, and melanomas have been reported. Generous sampling, particularly from solid areas, is recommended in older patients to exclude malignant transformation (Fig. 6.56).

Key Features of Mature Cystic Teratoma
- Cyst containing semi-liquid sebaceous material, hair
- Rokitansky protuberance in wall
- Lining by predominantly squamous epithelium
- Tissues representing all three germ cell layers
- Bilateral in 15% of cases

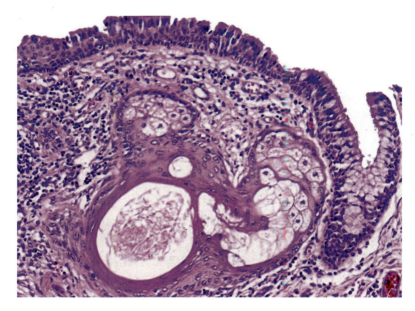

FIGURE 6.55 Mature cystic teratoma: Most cystic areas are lined by squamous epithelium and show ectodermal tissues such as hair follicles and sebaceous glands. Mucinous or ciliated columnar epithelia are evidence of endodermal differentiation (H&E, medium power).

Immature Teratoma

These tumors represent only 3% of teratomas, but are responsible for about 15% of ovarian malignancies in patients below 20 years of age. They form large mostly solid fleshy soft tumors (median 18 cm at laparotomy) with small cysts, necrosis, or hemorrhage. Microscopically, they are characterized by a disorderly mixture of mature and immature tissues derived from all three germ cell layers. The most common immature element is neuroepithelium which may form tubules or rosettes, glial tissue, cartilage, and other cell types (Figs. 6.57 and 6.58). In most cases, foci of mature teratoma are present. The final diagnosis should be deferred for permanent section, because extensive sampling is required to identify the foci of immature neural or other mesenchymal tissues, necessary for grading the neoplasm. Prognosis of immature teratomas correlates with the grade of primary tumor, as well as the presence and grade of peritoneal implants. Low-grade tumors confined to the ovary are treated with unilateral salpingooophorectomy, while grade 2,

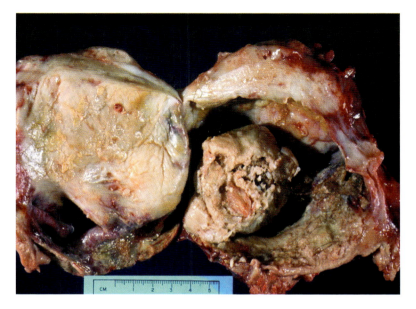

FIGURE 6.56 Carcinoma associated with mature cystic teratoma: This tumor, presenting in a postmenopausal patient, showed a classic cystic teratoma with sebaceous material and hair. The solid area, however, was almost completely involved by a well differentiated squamous cell carcinoma, the most common type of malignant transformation in mature cystic teratoma. From Ramzy I. Essentials of gynecologic and obstetric pathology. Norwalk: Appleton Century Crofts; 1983. p. 273. Used with permission.

grade 3, as well as more advanced lesions, are treated with surgical excision and chemotherapy. Peritoneal deposits are frequently encountered during surgery, but if they are glial, they almost always have a benign course.

Mature Solid Teratoma

These tumors have similar clinical features and gross appearance as immature teratomas, including the presence of neural tissue. However, they lack immature components and rarely show mitotic activity or necrosis. They follow a benign course.

Monomorphic Teratomas

Although these are rare neoplasms in the ovary, a brief discussion of some of them is warranted since they enter into the differential diagnosis of some common ovarian tumors.

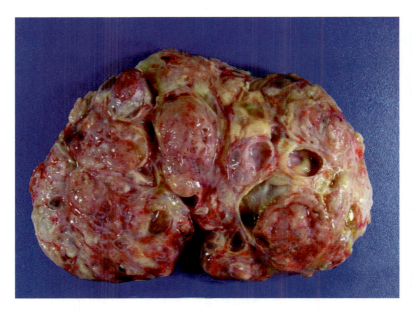

FIGURE 6.57 Immature teratoma: Note the bosselated outer surface of this mostly solid neoplasm.

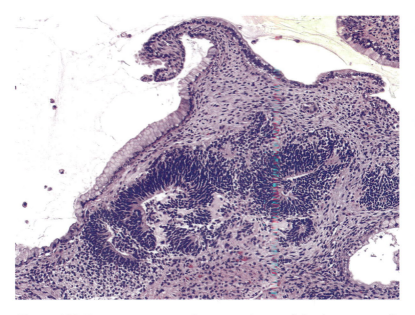

FIGURE 6.58 Immature teratoma: Immature tissues of the three germ cell layers are encountered. Neural tissue is usually the major component and is the basis for grading such tumors (H&E, low power).

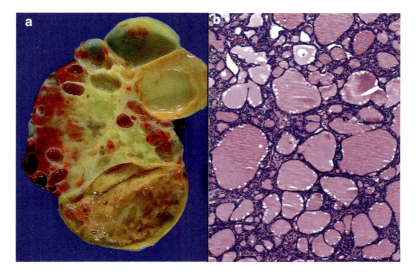

FIGURE 6.59 Struma ovarii: (**a**) A multinodular tumor, consisting of thyroid tissue with gelatinous-appearing translucent colloid material (H&E, low power). (**b**) Monodermal differentiation into thyroid tissue with follicles of variable sizes containing colloid (H&E, low power).

Struma ovarii shows features similar to normal thyroid or adenomatous nodules, rarely with papillae or hyperplasia. Although some tumors may have features of papillary or follicular carcinoma, almost all cases behave in a benign fashion. Struma ovarii may show calcium oxalate crystals, and immunoreactivity to thyroglobulin should help differentiating this neoplasm from Sertoli cell and granulosa cell tumors, carcinoid, yolk sac, clear cell, and other adenocarcinomas (Fig. 6.59).

Carcinoid is a solid brown to yellow neoplasm consisting of nests, acini, or trabeculae of neuroendocrine cells. These cells have round nuclei with salt-and-pepper chromatin pattern, cytoplasmic argentaffin granules, and stains positively for neuroendocrine markers such as chromogranin, serotonin, and 60% of cases stain positively for CD56.

Mucinous carcinoid is a rare neoplasm that, similar to other carcinoids, may be part of a teratoma or form a solid mass. The cells are similar to the classic carcinoid, with isolated goblet cells in a fibrous stroma, but argentaffin cells are rare. Mucinous carcinoid may be associated with mucinous carcinoma of the ovary; it should be differentiated from metastatic adenocarcinomas such as Krukenberg tumor, as discussed later.

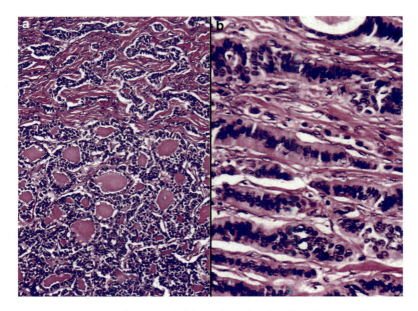

FIGURE 6.60 Strumal carcinoid: (**a**) Cords and trabeculae of neuroendocrine cells form separate nodules or are mixed with thyroid follicles. Within the tumor, the two components maintain their individual immunophenotype (H&E, low power). (**b**) Higher magnification illustrates the cords (H&E, medium power).

Strumal carcinoid is a benign neoplasm with microscopic features of struma and trabecular-insular carcinoid. It may present as a mass, hyperthyroidism, or carcinoid syndrome. It is immunoreactive to neuroendocrine markers such as chromogranin and synaptophysin, calcitonin, as well as thyroglobulin. The tumors often demonstrate transitional areas where the two cell populations merge into each other (Fig. 6.60). The individual cells in such cases retain their characteristic immunoprofiles.

Dysgerminoma

This neoplasm represents 1% of all germ cell tumors, but is the most common malignant tumor within that group, accounting for approximately 50% of all cases. It usually affects patients in the second or third decade, presenting most often as an adnexal mass, and rarely with primary amenorrhea. Dysgerminomas are typically solid, lobulated tan or gray/pink with a homogeneous cut surface, and are bilateral in about 15% of cases. Large tumors

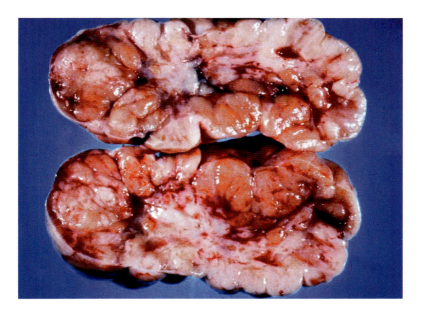

FIGURE 6.61 Dysgerminoma: A solid *grayish pink* tumor, resected from a 15 year old girl with no abnormal endocrine manifestations. The mass had a rubbery consistency and a fairly characteristic bosselated outer surface. The predominantly solid cut surface had the appearance of lymphoid tissue with an occasional area of hemorrhage and necrosis.

may show small cysts and hemorrhage. Histologic examination reveals a monotonous population of large cells with clear glycogen and lipid-rich cytoplasm, distinct cell boundary, and large central round vesicular nuclei (Figs. 6.61 and 6.62). The stroma contains a variable amount of T-lymphocytes, plasma cells, histiocytes, and eosinophils. About 15% of dysgerminomas demonstrate other germ cell components.

Differentiation from large cell lymphomas is usually feasible without the need for flow cytometry or immunohistochemistry. If necessary, however, a sample should be submitted for flow cytometric and cytogenetic studies at the time of frozen section. Although an occasional syncytiotrophoblast may be seen, cytotrophoblasts are lacking, unlike choriocarcinoma. Dysgerminomas lack the marked nuclear pleomorphism and hyperchromasia, dense cytoplasm, large numbers of syncytiotrophoblast-like cells, and positive cytokeratin that characterize embryonal cell carcinomas.

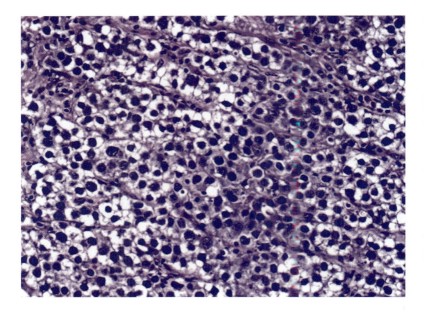

FIGURE 6.62 Dysgerminoma: Nests of large cells with abundant often clear glycogen rich cytoplasm. The large nuclei have prominent nucleoli and mitotic figures are frequent. Fibrous trabeculae infiltrated by a variable number of lymphocytes, surround the nests of germ cells (H&E, medium power).

Dysgerminomas are sensitive to chemotherapy. In most patients who desire to preserve fertility, a unilateral salpingooophorectomy with preservation of the contralateral ovary and uterus is sufficient, even in the presence of metastatic disease. If preservation of fertility is not a concern, a total abdominal hysterectomy and bilateral salpingooophorectomy is performed. In addition to the involved ovary, the contralateral ovary must be examined in all cases for any obvious gross lesions, capsular rupture, or adhesions.

Key Features of Dysgerminoma
- Solid bosselated gray pink mass with smooth surface and prominent vessels
- Cream gray or pink homogeneous cut surface
- Large tumors show hemorrhage, cysts, or necrosis
- Large germ cells with clear, pale glycogen, and lipid-rich cytoplasm
- Large vesicular nuclei
- Stroma with lymphocytes, plasma cells, and histiocytes
- Rare syncytiotrophoblast like cells
- Focal calcification

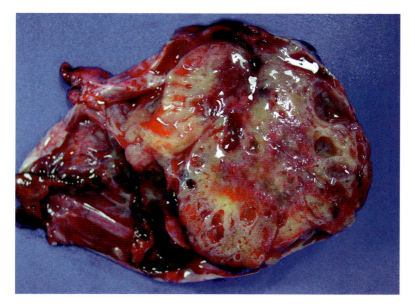

FIGURE 6.63 Yolk sac tumor: A 20 cm mass with a polymorphous cut surface in an 18 years old patient. The tumor shows extensive hemorrhage and necrosis. Microscopic examination revealed large foci of mature and immature teratomatous elements, in addition to the yolk sac pattern.

Other Malignant Germ Cell Tumors

Pure yolk sac tumor, embryonal carcinoma, and choriocarcinoma are rare in the ovary, comprising less than 10% of all malignant ovarian germ cell tumors. The majority present as mixed germ cell tumors, where more than one element can be identified.

Mixed germ cell tumors typically occur in women under 30 years of age. The tumors tend to be large and have a variable appearance, depending on the components. Extensive sampling is necessary and should include any gross areas of hemorrhage or necrosis, so as to identify possible immature neuroepithelium or malignant transformation in immature teratoma, as well as any highly aggressive elements, such as yolk sac, embryonal carcinoma, or choriocarcinoma (Figs. 6.63 and 6.64). If dysgerminoma is identified, inspection and/or biopsy of the contralateral ovary are indicated, since there is 5–10% likelihood of contralateral involvement. Poor prognostic indicators include large tumors (greater than 10 cm) and the presence of a major component (over one third)

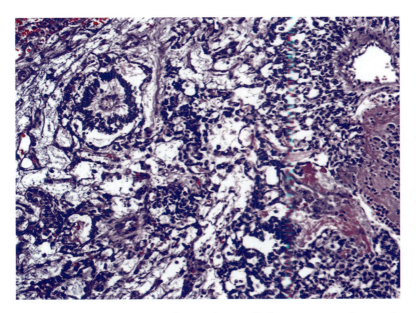

FIGURE 6.64 Yolk sac tumor: The neoplastic cells have scant cytoplasm and are arranged in nests, loose network of tubules within a loose stroma. A Schiller Duval body with a central vessel surrounded by a mantle of cuboidal cells within a glomerulus-like space is evident in the upper left corner (H&E, low power).

of embryonal carcinoma, choriocarcinoma, and/or high-grade teratoma. The different components, which rarely present in a pure form, are discussed below.

Embryonal carcinoma mostly presents with bleeding, precocious puberty, and a large pelvic mass. The tumor is predominantly solid, with smooth surface, a few cysts, necrosis, and hemorrhage. Histologically, nests and gland-like spaces are seen within primitive mesenchymal tissues and some syncytiotrophoblast cells.

Yolk sac tumor is usually a large (often 15 cm), bosselated cystic, gray to yellow tumor, with necrosis, hemorrhage, and myxoid gelatinous areas. Microscopically, branching cords, glandular spaces with papillary formations, and solid morules are seen. In about 25% of cases, Schiller–Duval bodies, with central blood vessel surrounded by a mantle of mesenchyme, covered by an outer layer of clear epithelial cells, are identified. The tumor is associated with high levels of α-fetoprotein and α (alpha)1-antitrypsin but not β (beta) hCG.

Choriocarcinoma is seen in 20% of mixed germ cell neoplasms, forming a large unilateral hemorrhagic and friable mass. A mixture of cytotrophoblast and syncytiotrophoblast cells with blood sinusoids is seen, associated with elevated serum hCG, as well as estrogenic or androgenic manifestations.

Gonadoblastoma affects children or young adults and is often associated with dysgenetic gonads, congenital anomalies, and hormonal manifestations. It is a combined tumor of germ cells surrounded by mantle of sex cord cells, hyaline material, and calcification. Dysgerminoma or other germ cell tumors may dominate the pattern.

METASTATIC TUMORS

The ovaries are the organs most commonly affected, within the female genital tract, by metastatic disease. Metastases to the ovary account for 6–7% of ovarian cancer found at surgery. Adenocarcinoma of the colon is the most frequent nongynecologic primary site of metastatic disease of the ovary, followed by breast and gastric carcinoma. Several mechanisms can be involved in the spread to the ovaries. Lymphatic spread is the most common mechanism for the spread from carcinomas of the colon, breast, stomach, and genitourinary tract, and such deposits often start at the hilum. Hematogenous dissemination occurs in late stage malignancies of many organs, while transluminal extension is the mechanism involved in the case of genital tract neoplasms, particularly the uterus. Transcelomic spread is primarily associated with abdominal viscera; tumors arising in pelvic organs spread by direct extension. Intraoperative consult is sought when an adnexal mass is encountered by the surgeon in the absence of prior history of malignancy. In addition, the primary tumor may be asymptomatic and too small to be detected, such as in the case of gastric carcinoma.

Gross and microscopic findings that suggest metastatic disease include bilateral or small unilateral tumors measuring <10 cm, extensive surface involvement, prominent lymphovascular invasion, and multinodular growth pattern. Other helpful criteria include small tumors confined to the medulla, sparing of follicular structures, and lack of transition from a benign component of a cyst wall to malignant. Raising the possibility of metastatic disease at the time of frozen section can lead to suboptimal debulking or understaging because metastatic tumors involving ovaries are treated more conservatively. However in many instances, especially in cases of poorly differentiated neoplasms, it is difficult to distinguish primary from metastatic malignancies. In such cases, the pathologist can make a diagnosis of cancer and defer determination of primary site for

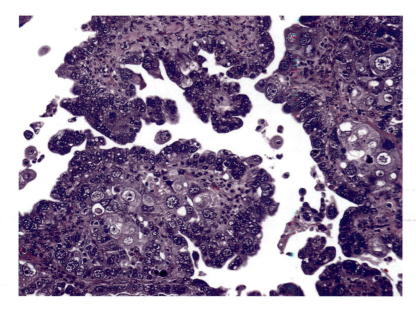

FIGURE 6.65 Effect of chemotherapy: A biopsy of serous carcinoma treated with adjuvant chemotherapy (Taxol-Carboplatin). The pleomorphic cells show degenerative changes in the cytoplasm and nuclei, with vacuolization and clumping of chromatin (H&E, medium power).

permanent sections and immunohistochemical stains. Another factor that may contribute to the difficulty in proper classification is the administration of adjuvant chemotherapy prior to surgery in the case of large neoplasms. The neoplastic cells in these cases show variable degrees of degenerative changes, such as cytoplasmic and nuclear vacuolization associated with bizarre nuclear morphology. Availability of previous material for review prior to frozen sections is invaluable (Fig. 6.65).

Key Features that Favor Metastases over Primary Ovarian Tumors
- Bilateral involvement or unilateral tumors measuring <10 cm
- Surface involvement
- Nodular growth
- Infiltrative growth pattern with desmoplastic stromal response
- Signet ring cell component
- Hilar involvement or lymphovascular invasion

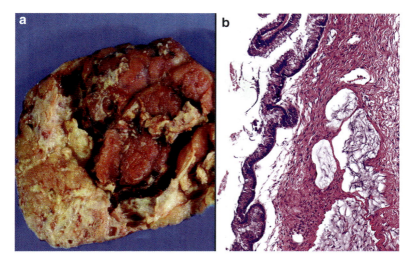

FIGURE 6.66 Metastatic carcinoma from colon: (**a**) The adnexal mass has a lobulated outer surface and shows extensive necrosis when opened. Other metastases may be associated with desmoplasia (H&E, low power). (**b**) Abundant mucin and malignant glands lined by tall columnar epithelium. Free mucin is seen dissecting the fibrous stroma (H&E, low power).

Metastatic mucinous carcinomas should be differentiated from primary mucinous ovarian carcinomas. Features that favor metastases include smaller, bilateral lesions with surface involvement. Metastatic carcinomas usually demonstrate a nodular pattern of invasion surrounded by zones of normal ovarian stroma. In contrast, primary ovarian mucinous carcinomas are large (>10 cm) unilateral lesions that typically have a smooth capsule with cystic and solid areas. Microscopically, transition from benign to borderline to an invasive component can be identified if an adequate number of slides is examined.

Colorectal cancer may present a particular clinical challenge, since ovarian metastasis is the first clinical evidence of the tumor in about 10% of cases, thus simulating primary ovarian cancer. It may also present as a large unilateral lesion that mimics mucinous cystadenocarcinoma or endometrioid carcinoma of the ovary, and the differentiation between these tumors may be difficult on the basis of histomorphology. The presence of dirty necrosis surrounded by "garlands" of markedly atypical mucinous cells, often with a cribriform arrangement, should raise the suspicion of metastatic colorectal carcinoma (Fig. 6.66).

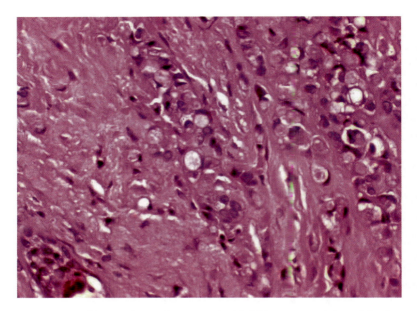

FIGURE 6.67 Metastatic mucinous carcinoid: This tumor, originated in the vermiform appendix (H&E, high power).

Appendiceal lesions, such as mucocele and mucinous neoplasms that are associated with pseudomyxoma peritoneii can also be confused with primary ovarian carcinoma. Mucinous variants of carcinoid tumors should be differentiated from metastatic adenocarcinomas such as Krukenberg tumor (Fig. 6.67).

Endometrioid like morphology is most commonly encountered in metastasis of colorectal origin, but other sites include stomach, gallbladder, bile ducts, appendix, pancreas, and the uterine cervix.

Breast cancer often metastasizes to the ovaries and is detected in about 10% of breast cancer patients at autopsy. Lobular carcinomas spread more frequently than ductal carcinoma, and usually the neoplastic cells are arranged as thin cords and single files. However, the neoplastic cells may form nests and diffuse sheets, with minimal pleomorphism and thus, can simulate granulosa cell tumors (Fig. 6.68). It is important to recognize that breast cancer patients are also at an increased risk for developing primary ovarian carcinoma, particularly in association with BRCA 1 and 2 mutations. Ovarian carcinoma in a patient with history of breast cancer is more likely to be a new primary. The diagnosis of primary ovarian carcinoma can be supported by features such as a large unilateral

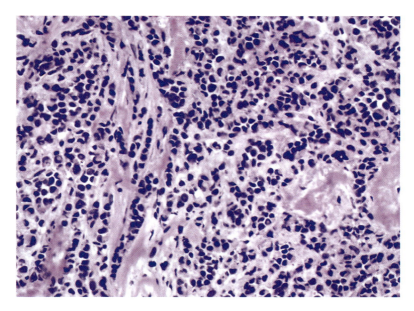

FIGURE 6.68 Metastatic carcinoma from breast: The neoplastic cells are small and occasionally retain the single file or a signet ring pattern (H&E, medium power).

lesion and a component of high-grade serous carcinoma, but in the absence of these features, it is hard to exclude metastasis and the final diagnosis should await permanent sections and immunohistochemical studies.

Metastases from lung carcinomas usually occur in patients with a known history, but in up to 16% of cases, the ovarian tumor is discovered first. Many of the metastatic lung carcinomas to the ovary present as unilateral lesions, but they often have multinodular growth and prominent vessel involvement that should alert the pathologist of possible metastatic disease.

Renal cell carcinoma can exhibit histologic patterns that mimic other tumors, including clear cell carcinoma of the ovary. However, clear cell carcinoma of the kidney rarely spreads to the ovary, usually retains the prominent sinusoidal vascular pattern, and has a uniform pattern and population of clear cells. In contrast, clear cell carcinoma of the ovary has diverse histologic patterns with areas of tubulocystic morphology. The neoplastic cells in ovarian clear cell carcinomas also show diverse morphology with an admixture of clear, cuboidal, hobnail, and flattened cells.

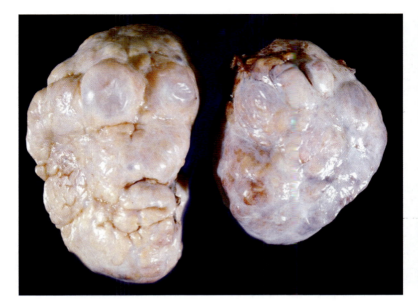

FIGURE 6.69 Krukenberg tumor: Both ovaries are enlarged, with a firm fibrous consistency. The ovarian shape is maintained. The patient had a 1 cm fissure which proved at autopsy to be a deeply infiltrating poorly differentiated gastric cancer. From Ramzy I. Essentials of gynecologic and obstetric pathology. Norwalk: Appleton Century Crofts; 1983. p. 296. Used with permission.

Cervical cancer can involve the ovaries, but in most cases, the cervical primary is evident and generally, these do not provide diagnostic problems. However, cervical adenocarcinomas can be small occult lesions that are first discovered as an ovarian mass. Adenoma malignum can simulate mucinous adenocarcinomas of the ovary, while endocervical adenocarcinoma can simulate endometrioid adenocarcinoma.

Peritoneal mesotheliomas may present a differential diagnostic challenge with ovarian carcinoma, particularly low-grade serous carcinomas, at the time of frozen section. It may require deferral for permanent sections and immunohistochemical stains. Peritoneal mesotheliomas often have papillary architecture but these papillae are less cellular and are lined by less pleomorphic cells. Prominent hyalinization can be seen in the cores of papillae of mesothelioma. In contrast, serous carcinomas have papillae that are more cellular and are lined by pleomorphic cells. Slitlike spaces and psammoma bodies are rarely seen in mesotheliomas.

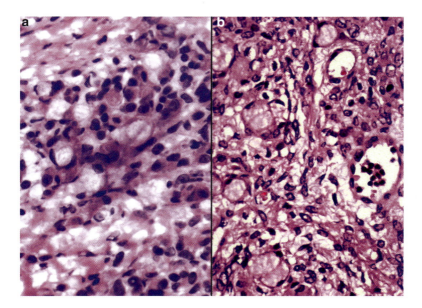

FIGURE 6.70 Krukenberg tumor: (**a**) Frozen section demonstrating signet ring cells with pleomorphic nuclei (H&E, medium power). (**b**) The few neoplastic cells may be masked by a prominent desmoplastic stromal response. The neoplastic cells should be differentiated from those of benign signet ring tumor depicted in Fig. 6.52 by their pleomorphic nuclei and presence of cytoplasmic mucin (H&E, medium power).

Krukenberg Tumor

This type of metastatic carcinoma accounts for 3–8% of all carcinomas metastatic to the ovaries. More than 80% are bilateral. Most Krukenberg tumors originate from the stomach; other sources include the breast, colon, appendix, pancreas, gallbladder, biliary tract, urinary bladder, and cervix. The ovaries are usually solid, asymmetrically enlarged, bosselated, and with firm white or yellow cut surface. The overall gross architecture is the preservation of the ovarian shape (Fig. 6.69). The tumor is predominantly composed of signet ring cells which may be sparse and easily missed on the frozen section. They are associated with plump spindled stromal cells which can mask the infiltrating neoplastic cells and can lead erroneously to the diagnosis of mesenchymal tumor (Fig. 6.70). A prominent tubular pattern may resemble lipid-rich Sertoli cell tumors, but is uncommon. Although benign signet ring cell tumors can be encountered,

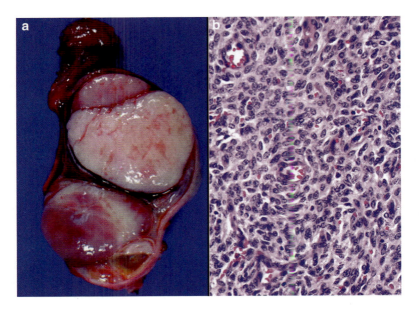

FIGURE 6.71 Metastatic endometrial stromal sarcoma: (**a**) A solid firm ovarian metastasis from a primary undifferentiated endometrial sarcoma. Low-grade tumors may also spread to the ovary and pelvic wall through venous channels, forming "worm-like" intravascular plugs. (**b**) Spindle low-grade endometrial stromal cells with slight nuclear pleomorphism and only a rare mitotic figure (H&E, medium power).

these are exceptionally rare, and are mucin negative, unlike true Krukenberg tumors (see Fig. 6.52). The solid fibrous like gross appearance may also be suggestive of metastatic soft tissue neoplasms or uterine sarcomas (Fig. 6.71), but the lack of epithelial elements on careful microscopic examination should establish the correct diagnosis, without the need for immunostains.

FALLOPIAN TUBE TUMORS

Primary neoplasms of the fallopian tube are rare, accounting for only 0.3–1.1% of all gynecologic malignancies. Secondary involvement, primarily by spread from ovarian or endometrial carcinomas, is much more common.

There is a higher rate of intraepithelial and invasive tubal carcinomas in women with BRCA1 and BRCA2 mutation. Also molecular and genetic data suggest that some of the ovarian or peritoneal serous epithelial cancers may originate in the distal fallopian tube epithelium. However, determination of primary site is not a consideration at the time of frozen section. Appropriate classification is done with permanent sections when the fallopian tubes and ovaries are extensively examined.

Almost all primary tubal neoplasms are malignant and discovered as an unexpected finding during laparotomy for an adnexal mass. Abnormal vaginal cytology is reported in 10–25% of advanced cases, and the tumor involves the peritoneum before seeding the ovary, resulting in positive peritoneal fluid cytology. Tubal carcinomas arise from müllerian epithelium and are morphologically similar to ovarian carcinomas. They can be of serous, endometrioid, and rarely transitional, clear cell, or squamous cell differentiation. Because of the rarity of carcinomas of the fallopian tube when compared to ovarian and endometrial carcinomas, strict criteria are required before classifying a tumor as primary in the fallopian tube. The main tumor mass must involve the tube; the uterus and ovaries are free of carcinoma, or contain significantly less tumor than the tube. Evidence of transition from benign tubal epithelium, to dysplastic/intraepithelial carcinoma to invasive carcinomas is helpful in determining the primary site, although the same transition may be seen in some cases of mucosal spread from uterine cancer. Ovarian carcinoma spreading to the tube involves the serosa and may spare the endosalpinx.

Benign conditions that should be considered in the differential diagnosis include salpingitis, endometriosis, tubal pregnancy, tubal torsion, pseudocarcinomatous hyperplasia, adenomatoid tumors, metaplastic papillary tumor, and leiomyomas.

RECOMMENDED READING

Baker P, Oliva E. A practical approach to intraoperative consultation in gynecological pathology. Int J Gynecol Pathol. 2008;27:353–65.

Barakat RR, Bevers MW, Gershenson DM, Hoskins WH, editors. MD Anderson Cancer Center and Memorial Sloan-Kettering Cancer Center Handbook of gynecologic oncology. 2nd ed. London: Martin Dunitz; 2002.

Berek JS, Neville HF, editors. Berek and Hacker's gynecologic oncology. 5th ed. Philadelphia, PA: Lippincott Williams & Wilkins; 2010.

DiSaia PJ, Creasman WT. Clinical gynecologic oncology. 7th ed. Philadelphia, PA: Moby-Elsevier; 2007.

Hart WR. Mucinous tumors of the ovary: a review. Int J Gynecol Pathol. 2005;24:4–25.

Hoskins W, Perez CA, Young RC. Principles and practice of gynecologic oncology. 3rd ed. Philadelphia, PA: Lippincott William & Wilkins; 2000.

Ismiil N, Ghorab Z, Nofech-Mozes S, et al. Intraoperative consultation in gynecologic pathology: a 6 year audit at a tertiary care medical center. Int J Gynecol Cancer. 2009;19:152–7.

Khonamornpong S, Settakorn J, Sukpan K. Mucinous tumor of low malignant potential ("borderline" or "atypical proliferative" tumor) of the ovary: A study of 171 cases with the assessment of intraepithelial carcinoma and microinvasion. Internat J Gynecol Pathol. 2011;30:218–30.

Kikkawa F, Ishikawa H, Tamakoshi K, et al. Squamous cell carcinoma arising from mature cystic teratoma of the ovary: a clinicopathologic analysis. Obstet Gynecol. 1997;89:1017–22.

Menzin AW, Rubin SC, Noumoff JS, LiVolsi VA. The accuracy of a frozen section diagnosis of borderline ovarian malignancy. Gynecol Oncol. 1995;59:183–6.

Michael CW, Lawrence WD, Bedrossian CW. Intraoperative consultation in ovarian lesions: a comparison between cytology and frozen section. Diagn Cytopathol. 1996;15:387–94.

Nucci MR, Oliva E. Gynecologic pathology. London: Elsevier Churchill Livingstone; 2009 (Volume in the series foundations in diagnostic pathology).

Obiakor I, Maiman M, Mittal K, et al. The accuracy of frozen section in the diagnosis of ovarian neoplasms. Gynecol Oncol. 1991;43:61–3.

Ramzy I. Signet-ring stromal tumor of ovary: histochemical, light and electron microscopic study. Cancer. 1976;38:166–72.

Robboy SJ, Anderson MC, Russell P. Pathology of the female reproductive tract. London: Churchill Livingstone; 2002.

Segal GH, Hart WR. Ovarian serous tumors of low malignant potential (serous borderline tumors). The relationship of exophytic surface tumors to peritoneal "implants". Am J Surg Pathol. 1992;16: 577–83.

Siedman JD, Kurman RJ, Ronnett BM. Primary and metastatic mucinous adenocarcinomas in the ovaries: Incidence in routine practice with a new approach to improve intraoperative diagnosis. Am J Surg Pathol. 2003;27:985–93.

Silva EG, Deavers MT, Malpica A. Patterns of low-grade serous carcinoma with emphasis on the nonepithelial-lined spaces pattern of invasion and the disorganized orphan papillae. Internat J Gynecol Pathol. 2010;29:507–12.

Snyder RR, Norris HJ, Tavassoli F. Endometrioid proliferative and low malignant potential tumors of the ovary. Am J Surg Pathol. 1988;12:661–71.

Stewart C, Brennan B, Hammond I, et al. Intraoperative assessment of ovarian tumors: a 5 year review with assessment of discrepant diagnostic cases. Int J Gynecol Pathol. 2006;25(3):216–22.

Taskiran C, Erdem O, Onan A, et al. The role of frozen section evaluation in the diagnosis of adnexal mass. Int J Gynecol Cancer. 2008;18:235–40.

Tempfer C, Polterauer S, Bentz EK, et al. Accuracy of intraoperative frozen section analysis in borderline tumors of the ovary: a retrospective analysis of 96 cases and review of the literature. Gynecol Oncol. 2007;107:248–52.

Usubutun A, Altinok G, Kucukali T. The value of intraoperative consultation (frozen section) in the diagnosis of ovarian neoplasms. Acta Obstet Gynecol Scand. 1998;77:1013–6.

Young R. From Krukenberg to today: the ever present problems posed by metastatic tumors in the ovary. Part II. Adv Anat Pathol. 2007;14:149–77.

# Chapter 7
Concluding Remarks

Intraoperative consultations should be requested only if results could impact immediate patient management. It is essential that the surgeon is aware of the use and limitations of intraoperative consultations. An accurate interpretation of frozen section depends on many critical steps that may be overlooked. The surgeon must provide adequate orientation of the specimen, details of clinical setting, and history, such as previous neoplasms, known gene mutations or family history, elevated tumor serum markers, prior use of neoadjuvant treatment or bilaterality, and specify questions to be addressed. The accuracy of frozen sections increases with clear communication of such pertinent clinical information. Errors in frozen section analysis can occur for a variety of reasons, including inadequate tissue sampling, technical problems that result in poor quality of microscopic preparations, or interpretative errors by the reporting pathologist. However, in most instances, intraoperative consultations in gynecologic specimens are accurate when determining the benign or malignant nature of a lesion, type of malignancy, status of resection margins or lymph nodes, and the extent and depth of involvement of a tumor. In cases that require an accurate mitotic count, determination of the degree of dysplasia, or when extensive sampling is necessary to establish the diagnosis, the role of intraoperative consultations is limited, and a definitive diagnosis can be deferred until the evaluation of permanent sections. In addition, the use of frozen sections in some situations may, in fact, alter the cytologic or architectural features necessary for establishing an accurate diagnosis. With this limitation in mind, the use of intraoperative consultation remains a highly sensitive and specific technique that plays a critical role in the management of gynecologic disease.

Index

A

Accuracy, frozen section, 2
Adenocarcinoma
  adenocarcinoma in situ (AIS), 83, 84
  cervix, 82–93
  clinical background and specimen handling, 39–40
  differential diagnostic considerations
    adenosis, 42, 50
    cauterization, endocervical margin, 91
    diagnostic problems, 91
    microglandular hyperplasia, 92
    progestational agents, 92
    prolapsed fallopian tube, 43, 51
    reactive atypia, 92
    tubal metaplasia, 91
  endometrium, 89–91, 120–128, 131
  glandular intraepithelial neoplasia, 83–84
  interpretation
    clear cell carcinoma, 41, 47
    endometriosis, 40, 42, 46
    morphology, 40
    neuroendocrine carcinomas, 41, 48, 49
  invasive, 84–85
  minimal deviation adenocarcinoma, 91
  mucinous adenocarcinoma, 85, 87–89
  vagina, 39–50
Adenocarcinoma in situ (AIS), 83, 84

Adenoid cystic carcinoma, 96, 97
Adenosarcoma, 107, 132, 141–142, 146, 150–151
Adenosis, 42, 50
Adnexal lesions, interpretation and differential diagnosis in, 162–163
Adult granulosa cell tumors, 196, 199
Aggressive angiomyxoma, 56, 57
Androblastoma, 202–204
Appendiceal lesions, 222

B

Basal cell carcinoma, 20, 29, 30
Benign and borderline clear cell tumors, 189
Benign disease, hysterectomy, 105
Biopsy
  cervical cone
    clinical background, 61
    conization impact, management, 69–70
    interpretation, 62
    limitations, conization, 62–69
    specimen handling, 62
  cervical punch, 59–60
  clinical background and specimen handling, 5–6
  interpretation and limitations, 6–7
  ovarian cancer
    omental and peritoneal, 160, 161
    wedge, 159–160
Breast cancer, 222, 223
Brenner tumors, ovary, 190–192

C

Carcinoid, 213
Carcinoma, endometrial
  clinical background, 119–120
  interpretation and differential
      diagnostic considerations
    adenocarcinoma, 123
    clear-cell carcinoma, 130
    differentiation, 126
    identification, 122–123
    key histologic features, serous
      carcinoma, 130
    mucin-rich/glycogen-rich
      neoplasms, 125
    secretory, 127
    serous papillary carcinoma,
      127–129
    sertoli-like pattern, 128
    villoglandular
      adenocarcinomas, 125, 129
  specimen handling, 120–122
Carcinosarcoma (malignant mixed müllerian tumor), 44, 97; 132, 143, 146–149
Cauterization, endocervical margin, 91
Cervical cancer, 224
  clinical background and types, 110–112
  interpretation, 112
  specimen handling, 112
Cervical cone biopsy, 61–70
  clinical background, 110–112
  conization impact, management, 69–70
  interpretation, 62
  limitations, conization
    CIN III and proper orientation, 66, 67
    diathermy effect, 68, 69
    embedding, 66, 67
    pseudoinvasion, 67, 68
    squamous metaplasia, 67
  specimen handling, 62
Cervical intraepithelial neoplasms (CIN), 64, 66, 68, 70, 74, 75, 85
Cervical malignancies, 73
Cervical punch biopsy, 59–60
Chemotherapy effects, 220
Choriocarcinoma, 219
CIN. *See* Cervical intraepithelial neoplasms (CIN)
Clear cell carcinoma
  adenocarcinoma, vagina, 41, 47
  endometrium, 130–131
  ovary, 189
  uncommon neoplasms, 97
  vagina, 33, 40, 41
Clear cell neoplasms, ovary, 188–189
Colorectal cancer, 221
Condyloma acuminatum, 18, 19, 38, 43
Condylomata acuminata, 38, 43
Conization
  impact on management, 69–70
  limitations of, 62, 66–70
Cystectomy, ovary, 158–159

D

Diathermy effect, 68, 69
Dysgerminoma, 208, 214–216

E

Embryonal carcinoma, 218
Embryonal rhabdomyosarcoma
  sarcomas and spindle cell lesions, 45, 52–54
  uncommon neoplasms, 98
Endocervical margin assessment, 71–73
Endometrial biopsy, 104–105
Endometrial carcinoma
  clinical background, 119
  interpretation and differential
      diagnostic considerations
    adenocarcinoma, 123
    clear-cell carcinoma, 130
    differentiation, 126
    identification, 122–123
    key histologic features, serous
      carcinoma, 130

mucin-rich/glycogen-rich neoplasms, 125
secretory, 127
serous papillary carcinoma, 127–129
sertoli-like pattern, 128
villoglandular adenocarcinomas, 125, 129
specimen handling, 120–122
Endometrial curettage and endometrial biopsy
clinical background, 104
interpretation and differential diagnostic considerations, 105
specimen handling, 104
Endometrial hyperplasia
clinical background, 115
differential diagnostic considerations, 116
interpretation, 115–119
specimen handling, 115
Endometrial polypectomy, 107–109
clinical background and specimen handling, 107
interpretation and differential diagnostic considerations, 107109
Endometrial stromal sarcoma, 140–149
Endometrioid adenocarcinoma, 40, 89–91, 113, 123–128, 185–188, 195, 198
variants, 125–128
Endometrioid adenofibroma, 186
Endometrioid like morphology, 222
Endometrioid tumors, 185–188
Endometriosis, 40, 46, 163, 165
Epithelioid smooth muscle tumor, 138–140, 142
Extramammary Paget disease, 24–27

F
Fallopian tube tumors, 226–227. *See also* Ovarian cancer
Fibroepithelial polyps, 54–56
Frankly invasive mucinous carcinomas, 183

G
Germ cell neoplasms
choriocarcinoma, 309
dysgerminoma, 214–216
embryonal carcinoma, 218
gonadoblastoma, 219
immature teratoma, 210–211
mature cystic teratoma, 208–210
mature solid teratoma, 211
mixed germ cell tumors, 217–218
monomorphic teratomas, 211–214
ovary, 208–219
yolk sac tumor, 218
Glandular intraepithelial neoplasia, 83–85
Glassy cell carcinoma, 96, 97
Gonadoblastoma, 219
Granulosa cell tumors, 194–199
Gross consult, 1, 2
Gutter lavages, 162

H
Hilus cell tumor, 205
Hyperplasia, endometrial
clinical background, 115
differential diagnostic considerations, 116–119
interpretation, 115
specimen handling, 115
Hysterectomy
for benign disease, 105–106
for cervical cancer
clinical background and types, 110–112
interpretation, 112
specimen handling, 112
for endometrial carcinoma, 119–131
clinical background, 119–120
interpretation and differential diagnostic considerations, 122–123
specimen handling, 119–122
for endometrial hyperplasia, 115–119
clinical background, 115

Hysterectomy (*cont.*)
   differential diagnostic considerations, 116
   interpretation, 115
   specimen handling, 115
  for sarcomas, 132–151
   clinical background, 132
   interpretation and differential diagnostic considerations, 133–138
   specimen handling, 132–133

I

Immature teratoma, ovary, 210–212
Intraoperative consultation
  accuracy, frozen section, 1
  reasons for, 1, 2, 6, 60, 103, 104
Intravenous leiomyomatosis, 141
Invasive adenocarcinomas, 82, 84–87, 93
Invasive cancer
  adenocarcinomas, 84–91
  squamous cell carcinoma, 13–17
   desmoplastic stromal response, 79
   differential diagnostic considerations, 80
   exophytic tumor, 77
   extensive necrosis, 82
   keratinization, 80
   small cell carcinoma, 81
   tumor diathesis, 79
   ulcerative lesion, 78
   verrucous carcinoma, 81
  squamous cell neoplasms, vagina, 40
Invasive implants, 178
Invasive squamous cell carcinoma, 13–16, 18, 36–37, 40, 77–82

J

Juvenile granulosa cell tumors, 189, 195, 196, 199

K

Krukenberg tumor, 224–226

L

Lavages, pelvic, peritoneal, 162
Leiomyoma
  intravenous, 141
  vs. leiomyosarcoma, 136
  myxoid, 137
  necrosis, 138
  symplastic, 136
  variants, 135
Leiomyosarcoma
  vs. leiomyoma, 134
  and other smooth muscle neoplasms, 133–142
  sarcomas and spindle cell lesions, 44
Leydig cell tumor, 204, 206
Loop electrosurgical excision procedure (LEEP), 59–61
Lymph node dissection in vulvar cancer, 20, 21
Lymph node sampling in ovarian cancer, 160, 162

M

Malignant germ cell tumors, other, 217–219
Malignant melanoma, 20–24, 27
Malignant mixed müllerian tumor, 190–191
Mature cystic teratoma, 208–211
Mature solid teratoma, 211
Metastatic malignant melanoma, 98, 99
Metastatic neoplasms, 29–30
Metastatic tumors
  appendiceal lesions, 222
  breast cancer, 222, 223
  cervical cancer, 224
  chemotherapy effects, 220
  colorectal cancer, 221
  endometrioid like morphology, 222–223
  Krukenberg tumor, 224–226

metastases from lung carcinomas, 223
in ovary, 219–226
peritoneal mesotheliomas, 224
renal cell carcinoma, 223
Metastatic vulvar neoplasms, 29–30
Microglandular hyperplasia, 92
Microinvasive carcinomas
of cervix, 61, 62, 69, 74, 76û77
key features, 77
superficial stroma, 76
Minimal deviation adenocarcinoma, 91
Mixed germ cell tumors, 217
Monomorphic teratomas, 211–214
Mucinous adenocarcinoma
ovarian cancer, 183–184
uterine cervix, 85–89
Mucinous carcinoid, 213
Mucinous cystadenofibroma, 178–180, 183
Mucinous cystadenoma, 179
Mucinous neoplasms, ovary, 178–184
Mucinous tumor of borderline malignancy, 181–182
Mucin-rich/glycogen-rich neoplasms, 125
Myomectomy, 106–107
clinical background, 106
specimen handling and interpretation, 106–107
Myxoid leiomyoma, 137

N

Neoplasm
cervical intraepithelial neoplasms (CIN), 74–75
clear cell, 189
condylomata acuminata, 38, 43
germ cell neoplasms (*see* Germ cell neoplasms)
leiomyosarcoma and other smooth muscle, 133–138
metastatic, 29–30
mucin-rich/glycogen-rich, 125
radical vaginectomy, 34–35, 38
uncommon neoplasms (*see* Uncommon neoplasms)
verrucous carcinoma, 41–42
Neuroendocrine carcinomas, 41, 48, 49, 93–95
adenocarcinoma, vagina, 40, 47–49
uterine cervix, 93–97
Noninvasive implants, 177
Nonneoplastic lesions, 163–167

O

Omental and peritoneal biopsies, 160, 161
Oophorectomy and salpingooophorectomy, 157–158
Ovarian and tubal specimens, 156
Ovarian biopsy, 159, 160
Ovarian cancer.*See also* Fallopian tube tumors
adnexal mass
interpretation and differential diagnosis, 162–163
non-neoplastic lesions, 163–166
surgery indications, 153–154
biopsy
omental and peritoneal, 160–162
wedge, 159–160
cystectomy
clinical background, 158–159
specimen handling and interpretation, 159
germ cell neoplasms
choriocarcinoma, 219
dysgerminoma, 214–217
embryonal carcinoma, 218
gonadoblastoma, 219
immature teratoma, 210–211
mature cystic teratoma, 208–211
mature solid teratoma, 211
mixed germ cell tumors, 217
monomorphic teratomas, 211–214
yolk sac tumor, 217–218
lymph node sampling, 160

Ovarian cancer. *See also* Fallopian tube tumorsadnexal mass (*cont.*)
  metastatic tumors
    appendiceal lesions, 222
    breast cancer, 222, 223
    cervical cancer, 224
    chemotherapy effects, 220
    colorectal cancer, 221
    endometrioid like morphology, 222–223
    Krukenberg tumor, 224–226
    metastases from lung carcinomas, 223
    peritoneal mesotheliomas, 224
    renal cell carcinoma, 223
  neoplasms, 155
  oophorectomy and salpingooophorectomy, 157–158
  pelvic, peritoneal and gutter lavages, 162
  risk assessing factors, 155
  sex cord and stromal tumors
    granulosa cell tumor, 191–200
    Hilus cell tumor, 205
    Leydig cell tumor, 205, 206
    Sertoli cell tumor (Pure), 204–205
    Sertoli–Leydig cell tumor (androblastoma), 202–204
    sex cord tumor with annular tubules (SCTAT), 206, 208
    signet ring stromal tumor, 206, 207
    Steroid cell tumor, 204–205
    theca cell tumor, 194, 199–203
  staging, adequate, 156
  surface epithelial tumors
    clear cell neoplasms, 188–189
    endometrioid tumors, 185, 187–188
    invasive peritoneal implants, 176–177
    malignant mixed müllerian tumor, 190, 193
    mucinous adenocarcinoma, 183–184
    mucinous cystadenofibroma, 178–180
    mucinous cystadenoma, 178–180
    mucinous tumor of borderline malignancy, 181–182
    noninvasive peritoneal implant, 176, 177
    peritoneal adenomucinosis (pseudomyxoma peritoneii), 185–186
    relative incidence, 166–168
    serous adenocarcinoma, 172–174
    serous borderline tumor, 172, 175
    serous carcinoma of peritoneum, 175, 177
    serous cystadenofibroma, 171
    serous cystadenoma, 169–171
    transitional cell (Brenner) tumors, 190
Ovarian torsion, 166
Ovary and fallopian tube, 153–227

P

Paget disease, 20, 24–27
Pelvic lymph-node resection
  clinical background, 112–113
  interpretation and differential diagnostic considerations, 113–115
  specimen handling, 113
Pelvic, peritoneal and gutter lavages, 162
Peritoneal adenomucinosis, 186
Peritoneal implants, 176–178
  invasive, 176–177
  noninvasive, 176, 177
Peritoneal mesotheliomas, 224
Polypectomy, endometrial
  clinical background and specimen handling, 107
  interpretation and differential diagnostic considerations, 107–109
Postradiation epithelial atypia, 38, 39, 44
Primary adenocarcinoma, vagina, 45

Prolapsed fallopian tube, 43, 51
Pseudoinvasion, 67, 68

R

Radical trachelectomy, 70–73, 82
  alternative techniques, 71
  clinical background, 70–71
  endocervical margin assessment, 71–73
  specimen handling, 71
Radical vaginectomy, 34–35, 38
Reactive atypia, 92
Renal cell carcinoma, 223
Rhabdomyosarcoma, 45–54

S

Salpingooophorectomy, 157–158
Sarcoma botryoides.See Embryonal rhabdomyosarcoma
Sarcomas
  clinical background, 44, 132–133
  interpretation and differential diagnostic considerations
    aggressive angiomyxoma, 56, 57
    Embryonal rhabdomyosarcoma, 45, 53–55
    endometrial stromal sarcoma, 140–151
    epithelioid smooth muscle tumor, 138–142
    Fibroepithelial polyps, 54–56
    leiomyosarcoma, 45
    leiomyosarcoma and other smooth muscle neoplasms, 133–136
    vaginal intraoperative consultations, 54
  specimen handling, 132
Secretory carcinoma, 127, 131
  endometrium, 130, 131
Serous borderline tumor, 172, 175
Serous carcinoma of the peritoneum, 175, 177
Serous cystadenocarcinoma, 173, 174, 177
Serous cystadenofibroma, 171
Serous cystadenoma, 169–171
Serous neoplasms, ovary, 169–177
Serous papillary carcinoma, 127–130
Sertoli cell tumor (Pure), 204–205
Sertoli–Leydig cell tumor (androblastoma), 202–204
Sex cord and stromal tumors
  granulosa cell tumor, 194–199
  Hilus cell tumor, 205
  Leydig cell tumor, 205, 206
  Sertoli cell tumor (Pure), 204–205
  Sertoli-Leydig cell tumor (androblastoma), 202–204
  sex cord tumor with annular tubules (SCTAT), 206, 208
  signet ring stromal tumor, 206, 207
  Steroid cell tumor, 204–205
  theca cell tumor, 194, 199–201
Sex cord stromal neoplasms, other, 204–208
Sex cord tumor with annular tubules (SCTAT), 206, 208
Signet ring stromal tumor, ovary, 206, 207
Smooth muscle tumor of uncertain malignant potential (STUMP), 134
Squamous cell cancer, vulvectomy
  clinical background and specimen types, 7–8
  interpretation and differential diagnostic considerations
    invasive squamous cell carcinomas, 13–15
    verrucous carcinoma, 16–19
    vulvar intraepithelial neoplasia (VIN), 11–14
  specimen handling, 8–10
Squamous cell carcinoma, 73–82
  cervical intraepithelial neoplasms (CIN), 74–75
  invasive squamous cell carcinoma
    desmoplastic stromal response, 79
    differential diagnostic considerations, 80

Squamous cell carcinoma (*cont.*)
  exophytic tumor, 77
  extensive necrosis, 82
  keratinization, 80
  small cell carcinoma, 81
  tumor diathesis, 79
  ulcerative lesion, 78
  verrucous carcinoma, 81
 microinvasive carcinomas
  key features, 77
  superficial stroma, 76
Squamous cell neoplasms, vagina
 clinical background, 33–34
 differential diagnostic
    considerations
  condylomata acuminata,
    38, 43
  postradiation epithelial atypia,
    38–40, 44
 interpretation
  fungating mass, surface
    ulceration and hemorrhage,
    39
  invasive, 40
  radical vaginectomy, 35–38
  vaginal intraepithelial
    neoplasia, 36–37
  verrucous carcinoma, 41–42
 specimen handling, 34
Squamous metaplasia, 67
Steroid cell tumor, 204
Strumal carcinoid, 214
Struma ovarii, 213
Surface epithelial neoplasms,
    other, 190–191, 193
Surface epithelial tumors,
    166–193
Symplastic leiomyoma, 136

T

Theca cell tumor and fibroma,
    199–208
Thecomatosis, 166, 167
Transitional cell tumors, ovary,
    190–192
Tubal metaplasia, 91

U

Uncommon neoplasms
 adenoid cystic carcinoma, 96, 97
 cervix, 93, 96–99
 clear cell carcinoma, 97
 embryonal rhabdomyosarcoma,
    97–99
 glassy cell carcinoma, 96, 97
 malignant melanoma, metastatic,
    97, 99
Uterine body
 endometrial curettage and
    endometrial biopsy
  clinical background, 104
  interpretation and differential
    diagnostic considerations,
    105
  specimen handling, 104
 endometrial polypectomy
  clinical background and
    specimen handling, 107
  interpretation and differential
    diagnostic considerations,
    107–109
 hysterectomy, benign disease,
    105–106
 hysterectomy, cervical cancer
  clinical background and types,
    110–112
  interpretation, 112
  specimen handling, 112
 hysterectomy, endometrial
    carcinoma
  clinical background, 119–120
  interpretation and differential
    diagnostic considerations,
    122–123
  specimen handling, 120–122
 hysterectomy, endometrial
    hyperplasia
  clinical background, 115
  differential diagnostic
    considerations, 116
  interpretation, 115–119
  specimen handling, 115
 hysterectomy, sarcomas
  clinical background, 132

interpretation and differential
diagnostic considerations,
133–141
specimen handling, 132–133
myomectomy
clinical background, 106
specimen handling and
interpretation, 106–107
pelvic lymph-node resection
clinical background, 112
interpretation and differential
diagnostic considerations,
114–115
specimen handling, 113
reasons, intraoperative
consultation, 103
uterine corpus specimens, 103–104
Uterine cervix
adenocarcinoma
differential diagnostic
considerations, 91–93
glandular intraepithelial
neoplasia, 83–85
invasive adenocarcinomas,
84–86
minimal deviation
adenocarcinoma, 91
mucinous adenocarcinoma, 85,
87, 88
cervical cone biopsy
clinical background, 61
conization impact,
management, 69–70
interpretation, 62
limitations of conization, 62–69
specimen handling, 62, 63
cervical malignancies, 73
cervical punch biopsy, 59–60
loop electrosurgical excision
procedure (LEEP), 60–61
neuroendocrine carcinomas, 94–95
radical trachelectomy
alternative techniques, 71–73
clinical background, 70–71
endocervical margin
assessment, 71
specimen handling, 71

squamous cell carcinoma
cervical intraepithelial
neoplasms, 74, 75
invasive squamous cell
carcinoma, 77–80
microinvasive carcinomas,
74–77
uncommon neoplasms, 97–99
Uterine corpus specimens, 103–104

V

Vagina
adenocarcinoma
clinical background and
specimen handling, 39–40
differential diagnostic
considerations, 42–43
interpretation, 40–41, 45–49
sarcomas and spindle cell lesions
clinical background, 44–45
interpretation and differential
diagnostic considerations, 45,
52–54
squamous cell neoplasms
clinical background, 33–34
differential diagnostic
considerations, 38–39, 43, 44
interpretation, 36–38
specimen handling, 34–35
Vaginal intraepithelial neoplasia, 36
Vaginectomy
for adenocarcinoma, 39–51
radical, 34–35, 38
for sarcomas and other spindle
cell lesions, 44–45, 52–57
for squamous cell neoplasms,
33–44
Verrucous carcinoma
cervix, 81, 97
squamous cell neoplasms, vagina,
38–39
vagina, 37, 41, 42, 81, 97
vulva, 17–19
vulvectomy, 17–18
Villoglandular adenocarcinomas,
83, 125, 130

Vulva
  biopsies
    clinical background and specimen handling, 5–6
    interpretation and limitations, 6–7
    intraoperative consultation, 3
    lymph node dissection, vulvar cancer, 20
    malignant melanoma, 20–29
    metastatic neoplasms, 29–30
  vulvectomy, squamous cell cancer
    clinical background and specimen types, 7–8
    interpretation and differential diagnostic considerations, 9–10
    specimen handling, 8–9
Vulvar intraepithelial neoplasia (VIN), 7, 11–14
Vulvectomy, squamous cell cancer
  clinical background and specimen types, 7–8
  interpretation and differential diagnostic considerations
    invasive squamous cell carcinomas, 13–16
    verrucous carcinoma, 17–19
    vulvar intraepithelial neoplasia (VIN), 11–13
  specimen handling, 9–10

W

Warty (condylomatous) carcinoma, 19
Wedge biopsy, 159–160

Y

Yolk sac tumor, 218

Printed in the United States of America